Table of Contents

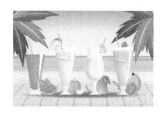

Introduction

Cancer is scary. Millions of people get diagnosed every year, and it's hard to find someone who hasn't been affected by the disease in some way. In America, the most common types of cancer are skin, lung, prostate, breast, and colorectal. While there isn't anything you can do to *guarantee* you'll never get cancer, there are things you can do to significantly lower your risk. Every expert will recommend exercise and a healthy diet. If you're reading this book, you want to know how smoothies fit into the picture.

Smoothies are a blend of ingredients like fruit, veggies, and a liquid of some kind. While the smoothies you buy at chain stores are often packed with sugar, which kind of negates the health benefits of the other ingredients, homemade smoothies can easily be part of a healthy diet that lowers your risk for cancer. I'll walk you through the best ingredients, how to buy and prep them, and how to choose the perfect blender. I'll also explore the reasons why smoothies are so good for cancer prevention, as well as why they're helpful *during* cancer treatment.

Nutrition is very important at any time of your life, but during cancer treatment, it's especially essential. Your body is worn down and side effects can make it hard to eat regular food. Smoothies fill in the gaps. This book has a chapter dedicated specifically to smoothies designed to help reduce symptoms like nausea and heartburn. It also includes a chapter of high-protein smoothies, because protein is very important during treatment. The rest of the chapters are labeled as either for cancer prevention or for both prevention and during treatment.

Whether you're a big fan of fruit-based smoothies or want to incorporate more greens into your diet, this is the book for you. If you need to increase your protein during treatment or fight side effects like nausea and fatigue, you'll find smoothies here, too. There's also chapters for tea and coffee-based smoothies, and smoothies you can have for dessert. All include lots of ingredients shown to have anti-cancer properties, so they can be part of a diet designed to protect you against disease. While this book isn't a substitute for medical advice from a professional, it can be a part of a healthy lifestyle and give you dozens of ideas for smoothies for every time of the year and any time of day.

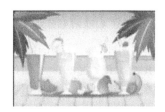

Chapter 1: Why Smoothies?

What is it about smoothies that make them great? While smoothies can easily become unhealthy with the wrong ingredients, with the *right* ones they have a lot of benefits. In this chapter, I break down why smoothies are effective at reducing your risk for cancer, and why they're a great food choice for people going through cancer treatment. I also go over a number of the best anti-cancer ingredients for smoothies and the research that shows why.

Why smoothies are good for cancer prevention

When it comes to doing everything you can to stay healthy and prevent cancer, why drink smoothies? There are three reasons: they're a great way to get in fruit and veggies; they're a source of nutrients; and they're easy and customizable.

Get more fruits and vegetables

Studies show that a diet rich in fresh fruit and vegetables lowers your risk for cancer. It can be very hard to get in the right amount, however, especially vegetables. Smoothies are a great way to eat more and even mask certain ingredients you aren't too fond of, like dark leafy greens.

Get essential nutrients

The staples of smoothies - fruits and vegetables - are packed with nutrients shown to lower one's risk for cancer. Fiber is an especially important one. Lots of fruits and veggies are high in antioxidants, as well, which have been shown to reduce inflammation, inhibit cancerous cell growth, and more. In smoothie form, you can get these nutrients all at once, and don't have to figure out ways to make a plate of spinach taste good.

Smoothies are easy to make and easy to tweak

To make a smoothie, you just pour a liquid like water, milk, or juice into a blender and add the rest of the ingredients. With a good blender, blending is fast and produces consistent results. It's the perfect breakfast or snack when you're busy and need something nutritious. Smoothies are also extremely adaptable, and you can switch out fruits, vegetables, and other add-ins like chia seeds to make endless combinations. It's hard to get bored with smoothies when you're tweaking flavors, so you can keep good cancer-fighting nutrition in your life for the long-term.

Why smoothies are good for cancer patients

You know the general benefits of smoothies, but why are they a great choice for people with cancer? There are four main reasons: they're easy; they provide good nutrition; they're a great way to get in calories; and they can ease common side effects from treatment.

- **They're easy**

When you have cancer, life changes significantly. It can seem like everything has been put on hold. Treatment and recovery are both often brutal and hard on your body, so you have little to no energy or motivation. Who wants to cook? Smoothies are way easier than preparing a whole meal. There's very little work involved beyond maybe some chopping. The blender does all the work.

- **They're nutritious**

Eating can be really hard when you're going through cancer treatment. Nausea and other stomach symptoms are common, so getting enough nutrition is a big concern. Smoothies are the perfect vehicle for fast, easy nutrition that's easy on the body. When you use the right ingredients (all the smoothies in this book are full of them), smoothies can help you get in the vitamins and minerals you need to function and heal properly. For this reason, many doctors and dietitians advocate for smoothies during treatment.

- **They're high-calorie**

Your body needs calories to work its best, and when you're going through something as traumatic as cancer treatment, your body needs all the calories it can get. Unfortunately, eating can be unpleasant, as I've mentioned, and weight loss is a common side effect during treatment. A smoothie can get you the calories you need in a more appealing package, so you're able to maintain a healthy weight.

- **They ease symptoms**

During treatment, a number of side effects are common, like nausea and loss of appetite. Mouth symptoms also occur a lot, because of the treatment breaking down the cells found there. Food can even taste metallic, and chewing is often uncomfortable. Smoothies can help with all these issues. They are easier to consume when you aren't that hungry, and can be made with nausea-relieving ingredients like ginger. They are also smooth and cool, which can ease mouth pain and dryness.

Best anti-cancer smoothie ingredients

You're going to get a lot of smoothie recipes in this book that contain ingredients known for their possible anti-cancer properties. Let's list a bunch of those ingredients right now, and explore the evidence and research that's been done. There are many other foods that may be good for preventing cancer and easing side effects of treatment, (i.e. tomatoes) but I'm going to discuss the ones that work in smoothies.

Fruits

Pretty much all fruits contain nutrients shown to prevent and fight cancer, especially antioxidants. However, these are the ones that are especially good. They will make repeat appearances in the recipes in this book.

Red grapes

Red grapes are packed with antioxidants and cancer-fighting nutrients. The skin contains resveratrol, which lab studies suggest may slow or even prevent tumor growth in the liver, stomach, skin, colon, breast, and more. Red grapes also have quercetin, a flavonoid that may slow down cancer growth.

Berries

Berries like blueberries, blackberries, and so on have lots of very powerful antioxidants. These could help prevent the development of free radicals. Animal studies with breast cancer, and blueberries and black raspberries have shown good results. More research is needed to determine how exactly berries impact cancer in humans, but the fruits are definitely beneficial in some way.

Apples

Apples are a good source of phytochemicals, which include quercetin and triterpenoids. These are antioxidants. Apples also contain polyphenols, which may prevent inflammation. Early research shows the polyphenols might inhibit cancerous cell growth. One specific type of polyphenol, phloretin, inhibited growth of breast cancer cells in a study from 2018. Organic unsweetened applesauce is also a good choice for smoothies.

Cherries

Cherries, both sweet and tart, also contain phytochemicals. Tart cherries in particular may have better cancer-fighting properties, however. In lab studies, the antioxidants in tart cherries reduced cancer growth. The amount of antioxidants in tart cherry juice is similar to fresh cherries, so cherry juice is also a good smoothie ingredient.

Cranberries

Cranberries are full of fiber and vitamin C, as well as a specific compound shown to reverse and slow the development of gum disease. Why does this matter? People with gum disease have a significantly higher risk of getting pancreatic cancer, which is one of the most common types of cancer in the United States. Eating cranberries or drinking organic cranberry juice is a great way to protect your gum health, and as a result, your pancreatic health.

Watermelon

In addition to being a delicious source of hydration, which is very important for cancer patients, watermelons have a lot of lycopene, a type of phytochemical. Lycopene is most recognized in tomatoes, but studies show that the lycopene in watermelon is just as well-absorbed. In fact, you could absorb more lycopene from watermelon than raw tomatoes.

Papaya and mango

Papaya is full of lycopene and carotenoids, which are known to fight free radical cells. A lab study done on papaya leaf extract showed it fought against lab-grown tumors. The extract also boosted certain chemicals that strengthen the immune system.

Mango, which is probably the more popular tropical fruit (at least here in the United States), contains antioxidants and polyphenols. In a study from 2014, researchers exposed breast cancer cells to these polyphenols and found that they significantly decreased cell growth. Mango has also shown a positive effect on inflammatory bowel disease and subsequently colon cancer.

Vegetables

For a really healthy smoothie, vegetables are a must-use ingredient. They add really potent antioxidants and other nutrients like fiber. While not always as tasty as fruit, their flavors can be hidden, if necessary, and their sweetness enhanced with other ingredients.

Leafy greens

A true superfood, it's no surprise that leafy green veggies may have cancer-fighting properties. These veggies are packed with antioxidants like lutein and beta-carotene. According to the American Institute for Cancer Research, there's lab research suggesting that the carotenoids in dark leafy greens can halt cancer growth, specifically in breast, skin, lung, and stomach cancer. Leafy greens include:

- Spinach
- Kale
- Swiss chard
- Collard greens
- Beet greens
- Romaine lettuce

Carrots

This veggie contains antioxidants like luteolin, which in lab studies demonstrated anti-cancer properties, and beta-carotene. Beta-carotene has been studied for its possible ability to guard cell membranes and slow cancer cell growth. Other phytochemicals in carrots may protect against specific cancers like breast, mouth, and stomach cancer.

Beets

This vibrant vegetable contains betalain, an antioxidant shown to have anti-cancer effects. Research on animals suggests it can prevent the formation of carcinogens, substances that can lead to cancer, and boost production of your immune cells.

Sweet potato

Sweet potatoes are bright orange, and the reason for that is compounds known as carotenoids. These are essentially antioxidants, and in lab studies, they control cell growth and help reduce a person's risk for cancer. Sweet potatoes are also a good source for nutrients like potassium and fiber.

Wheat grass

A health food powerhouse, wheat grass is full of antioxidants and may be able to lower cancer risk, and also help with the side effects of chemotherapy. How? During chemotherapy, patients might experience myelotoxicity, which harms the immune system. Wheat grass juice reduces that myelotoxicity, according to a study done with patients going through breast cancer and chemotherapy.

Spirulina

This blue-green algae is packed with healthy nutrients like vitamin E and antioxidants. It's also a popular source for plant proteins. According to one study, spirulina offered protection against oral cancer among people who chew tobacco.

Spices, seeds, nuts, and herbs

Fruits and veggies may make up the bulk of a smoothie, but spices, seeds, nuts, and herbs can add essential nutrients and flavor. A little goes a long way, so it's also an affordable way to use ingredients. I've included green tea and coffee in this section, even though they are beverages, because tea leaves are more like herbs, and coffee beans are seeds. As with the section before, there are many other spices, seeds, nuts, and herbs that show cancer-preventing properties, but we're going to describe the ones used frequently in smoothies.

Turmeric

An ingredient most commonly found in curries, turmeric contains curcumin, a substance with antioxidant and anti-inflammatory traits. According to research from the American Cancer Society, curcumin might prevent the development of cancer cells and shrink tumors. Research is still in the relatively early stages, but turmeric seems to have the most fighting power against bowel, stomach, skin, and breast cancer.

Cinnamon

A warming spice, cinnamon has been used medicinally for centuries. It contains antioxidants like polyphenols, and acts as an anti-inflammatory. According to studies, it may help reduce cancerous cell growth and even kill them.

Ginger

There isn't much research on ginger and cancer, though scientists are focused on its effects on ovarian cancer right now. In at least one study with mice, ginger halted cancer growth. However, the main reason we've included ginger is because of its long history as an ingredient that eases nausea. Some studies support that ginger can even help patients after chemotherapy, but again, the research is still new. Some people are adamant that ginger is a lifesaver when it comes to nausea, while others aren't as affected. You'll have to try it for yourself.

Flaxseed

Flaxseed contains lots of fiber, magnesium, and thiamin. It also has omega-3 fatty acids, which possess anti-inflammatory effects. Since inflammation is believed to have a connection to cancer, flaxseed could have benefits. There's also research that shows a connection to foods high in fiber (like flaxseed) and a lower risk for colorectal cancer. Research is still in its early stages, but flaxseed may reduce cancer cell growth in men with prostate cancer. You should also know, however, that flaxseed might interfere with the absorption of medication, so talk to your doctor before using the ingredient.

Chia seeds

These little seeds are full of nutrients like fiber, protein, and antioxidants. According to the Memorial Sloan-Kettering Cancer Center, the seeds may also have anti-cancer qualities. Because of the fatty acids and their anti-clotting properties, chia seeds may increase your risk of bleeding. Talk to your doctor before incorporating them into your smoothies.

Sunflower and pumpkin seeds

Full of nutrients like thiamin, vitamin E, and selenium, sunflower seeds are antioxidant-rich. Vitamin E in particular may protect the body from damage caused by free radicals, so it lowers your risk for cancer. Specific studies have shown that sunflower seed oil may help reduce risk of breast cancer. Pumpkin seeds have comparable benefits and nutrients like manganese, magnesium, and phosphorus. Sunflower seeds are slightly higher in phytosterols, which studies show can help fight breast, lung, liver, stomach, prostate, and ovarian cancer.

Tree nuts

Recent research suggests that cashews and other tree nuts have positive effects on colon cancer patients. Researchers aren't sure why exactly, though it may be because of the fact that cashews decrease insulin resistance, so more studies are needed. Like most nuts, cashews are healthy for other reasons, like their high antioxidant count.

Walnuts have lots of polyphenols, compounds that we're mentioning a lot in this section. A study from Marshall University showed that eating two ounces of walnuts per day for two weeks inhibited breast cancer growth. Other tree nuts include pistachios, macadamia nuts, and pecans.

Tea

We've known that green tea is a powerful antioxidant for a long time. Antioxidants are very important in preventing cancer, specifically free radical damage. Free radicals, while a normal part of a healthy body, can cause horrendous damage when there are too many. These free radicals damage parts of a cell, including its DNA, which may lead to cancer. Lab research and animal research shows that antioxidants can help counter that damage. Research also shows that a specific chemical known as epigallocatechin-3 gallate fights against an enzyme that causes cancer growth. 1 cup of green tea has between 100-200mg of that e3g chemical.

What about other types of tea? All teas have antioxidants, but in varying amounts. Black tea, which is caffeinated, has much lower amounts. Studies show it might have a positive effect on lung, prostate, and bladder cancers. Oolong tea is somewhere between green and black tea in terms of antioxidants. White tea is comparable to green tea, though it has different amounts of polyphenols. The benefits of herbal tea, which isn't true tea but infusions of herbs, fruit, and/or spices, vary. Depending on the ingredients, herbal tea definitely can have anti-cancer properties.

Coffee

The connection between cancer and coffee has been explored for decades, and research is still unclear. However, recent studies show that coffee may reduce the risk of certain cancers like breast and liver cancer. There are hundreds of active compounds in coffee, including polyphenols, which have been shown to fight cancer in a variety of ways. For the purposes of this book, we're using coffee more as a vehicle for other more solid anti-cancer ingredients than as a beneficial addition unto itself.

Parsley

This leafy herb contains antioxidants, specifically in the form of quercetin, a plant pigment. This compound has been shown to reduce cancer cell growth. Parsley is also rich in another compound, a flavone called apigenin, and can stop cancer cells from reproducing. Because of studies that show parsley might interact negatively with chemotherapy drugs, it should only be used as a preventative, and not during treatment.

Whole grains

Whole grains are packed with nutrients studied for their anti-cancer properties. These include polyphenols, saponins, and phytic acid. Whole grains are also full of fiber, which has been shown in studies to reduce the risk of colon cancer, breast cancer, and gastric cancer. Examples of whole grains used in smoothies include:

- Oats (instant and steel-cut)
- Quinoa (raw or cooked)
- Barley (cooked)

Honey

Honey has been researched a lot for potential anti-cancer effects, and studies show it has anti-inflammatory, antioxidant, and antitumor properties. While researchers are still searching for more answers, there's lots of evidence to suggest that honey can help prevent cancer. Different types of honey may have different effects. Manuka honey, a honey produced in New Zealand is especially interesting to many people, since it has a higher antioxidant count than other types. At least one study showed manuka honey inhibited cancer cell growth. Because manuka honey is so expensive, I'm sticking with regular honey in this book.

Dairy

In general, I avoid dairy in anti-cancer smoothies because dairy can be inflammatory. I use nut milks in these smoothies, but that doesn't mean all dairy is off-limits. There are two specific products used in the recipes:

Greek yogurt

A good source of protein and nutrients important during cancer treatment recovery, Greek yogurt is a great addition to anti-cancer smoothies. Some of these nutrients include calcium, vitamin B12, and probiotics, which can help restore a healthy balance of gut bacteria. Your gut health is extremely important, since it dictates the state of your immune system.

In this book, I use plain yogurt a lot, which has much less sugar than flavored varieties. Even then, depending on the brand, the nutritional info varies, so your specific smoothie might contain different calories, protein, fiber, etc., than the information given in the recipes.

Cottage cheese

Cottage cheese, which is made from curds of pasteurized cow's milk, is a good source of protein and nutrients like B6 and potassium. It can be used as an alternative to nonfat Greek yogurt for higher-protein smoothies.

Resources to check out

If you're interested in digging into the science yourself, here's a very abbreviated list of the types of resources I've investigated for my research on anti-cancer and cancer treatment nutrition:

American Institute for Cancer Research

https://www.aicr.org/

Cancer Research UK. (n.d.). *The immune system and cancer*. [online] Available at: https://www.cancerresearchuk.org/about-cancer/what-is-cancer/body-systems-and-cancer/the-immune-system-and-cancer

Donaldson, M. (2004). Nutrition and cancer: A review of the evidence for an anti-cancer diet. *Nutrition Journal*, 3(1).

Freitas, R. and Campos, M. (2019). Protective Effects of Omega-3 Fatty Acids in Cancer-Related Complications. *Nutrients*, 11(5), p.945.

Kampa, M., Nifli, A., Notas, G. and Castanas, E. (2007). Polyphenols and cancer cell growth. *Reviews of Physiology, Biochemistry and Pharmacology*, pp.79-113.

Mendes, E. (2018). *Coffee and Cancer: What the Research Really Shows | American Cancer Society*. [online] Cancer.org. Available at: https://www.cancer.org/latest-news/coffee-and-cancer-what-the-research-really-shows.html

Ramprasath, V. and Awad, A. (2015). Role of Phytosterols in Cancer Prevention and Treatment. *Journal of AOAC International*, 98(3), pp.735-738.

Yuan, J. (2013). Cancer prevention by green tea: evidence from epidemiologic studies. *The American Journal of Clinical Nutrition*, 98(6), pp.1676S-1681S.

www.cancer.ca. (n.d.). *Nutrition for people with cancer - Canadian Cancer Society*. [online] Available at: https://www.cancer.ca/en/cancer-information/cancer-journey/living-with-cancer/nutrition-for-people-with-cancer/?region=on

World Cancer Research Fund & American Institute for Cancer Research (AICR). (2007). Food, Nutrition, Physical Activity, and the Prevention of Cancer: A Global Perspective. Washington,

DC: American Institute for Cancer Research (AICR). Retrieved from: http://www.dietandcancerreport.org/.

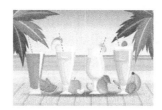

Chapter 2: Smoothie Blenders 101

To create your smoothies with the ingredients I've discussed, you need a blender. There's a huge range of options out there, but they aren't interchangeable in terms of quality. Getting the right blender matters. Poor-quality blenders won't do a good job of blending properly, so you'll end up with chunks or weird textures. They also won't last very long with daily use. To find the right one for your needs, there are four features you need to look at: power, blades, the jug, and the price. Let's break it down.

Power

Many smoothie makers believe the power of a blender is the most important feature, which makes sense. Without the right amount of power, you won't be able to blend everything you want, like ice and frozen fruit. A weak blender will also wear out much faster than a powerful one. Websites like *Spruce Eats* and *Taste of Home* recommend *at least* 500 watts for a smoothie blender. For the purpose of this book, I'm recommending a blender with a higher wattage, however, because of how often you'll want to make the recipes. Generally, the higher the wattage, the faster and more effective the blender will be at blending everything to a smooth consistency.

Blades

After power, blades are the most important part of a blender. You could have a high-wattage blender, but with the wrong blades, your smoothies won't turn out as good as they could. The best blades will be durable and able to handle tasks like blending ice, root vegetables, and other tough ingredients. You'll often see blenders advertising features like multiple rows of blades, which can be good for pureeing fibrous ingredients like kale. Be sure to pay close attention to the materials used, however, before choosing a blender. High-grade stainless steel is a great choice. You'll also want the blades to be removable, which is pretty standard these days, but there are still some with "fixed" blades. Don't get any of those.

The jug

The container is where all your ingredients actually go and get blended up. Most of the time, blender jugs are made of thick plastic. Be sure it's BPA-free and dishwasher-safe, if you don't want to hand-wash the jug every time. A leak-proof lid is another great feature to consider. You should also check out the jug size, which lets you know how many servings the blender can make. Small blenders make single servings around 1-2 cups, while big ones can make enough smoothies for 4 or more people. If you're the only one drinking a smoothie, a smaller blender is a good idea. With a larger one, you'll end up with leftovers, and smoothies don't taste the same after a stay in the fridge. A smaller blender will also take up less space on your counter.

The price

You can find a great smoothie blender no matter what your budget is. Smoothie blenders range significantly in price, from under $100 to $400 or more, if there are extras like travel cups, etc., included with your purchase. Brand name often plays into the price, so there may not be a huge difference in quality between a blender that's $100 and one that's $150. Look at reviews to see what real people are saying before making your selection.

Other features

The four features I mentioned above are the most important, but blenders often come with additional qualities that you might care about. These can include manual speed control, tampers, add-ons like travel cups, and so on. Many blenders have set speed modes, but a lot of people like manual speed control. Why? With manual control, you can gradually speed up the blending process, which ultimately creates evenly-blended smoothies free from air bubbles, which can lead to chunkiness. A tamper also helps with blending; it lets you push down larger chunks to the bottom of the jug for better circulation. With blenders that don't have a tamper, you'll be tempted to use a wooden spoon or other tool, and those can hurt the blades.

The last feature, extra products like travel cups and lids, are basically convenient goodies that can make an expensive purchase more worth it. Depending on the brand, however, a 12-piece set for cheap probably means the products aren't that high-quality, or the company wouldn't be practically giving them away.

Most popular brands

What smoothie blender brands are people buying? There are quite a few to know about:

- KitchenAid - reliable brand with affordable options
- NutriBullet - sleek design w/ mid-range price
- Oster- wide range of prices
- Breville - wide range of prices and sizes
- Ninja - lots of budget options
- Vitamix - the mother of blenders and pricey

How to blend the perfect smoothie

Equipped with a good blender and your ingredients, you are ready to make a smoothie. However, you can't just throw in the ingredients willy-nilly and expect perfect results. There is a method to the madness. Take a look at the graphic below for the proper order of ingredients:

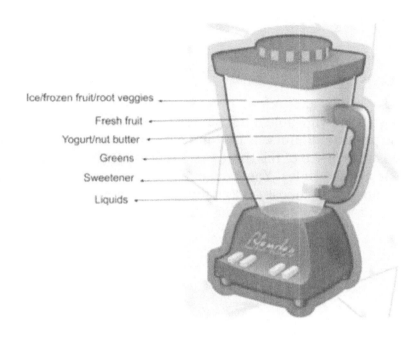

Ice/frozen fruit/root veggies
Fresh fruit
Yogurt/nut butter
Greens
Sweetener
Liquids

How big will a smoothie turn out? It depends. I generally try to keep the smoothies around 2 cups or so, with 1 cup or so of a liquid or yogurt base. Other ingredients like fruit or vegetables add another cup for a total of 2 cups.

Washing your blender

Cleaning up after a smoothie is never fun. However, it can be done really quickly. Simply fill your dirty blender halfway with hot water and add a teeny bit of dish soap. For extra cleaning power, squirt in a little lemon juice. Attach the blender back to the motor base, and blend for 10 seconds or so. This gets every corner really soaped up, and the power of the spinning blades and moving water breaks down smoothie residue. After blending, pour out the water and rinse the jug really well. Every once in a while, you will want to do a deeper clean where you actually remove the blades, wash them by hand, and make sure there isn't any gunk hanging out.

Other good equipment

You don't need a lot of equipment beyond a blender to make smoothies. In fact, I think you really only need three other things: freezer bags, ice cube trays, and a little food processor.

Freezer bags

For freezing fruits and vegetables, you need bags meant for the freezer. Gallon Ziploc bags work just fine. They are designed to keep out freezer burn and they're cheap.

Ice cube trays

Smoothie recipes occasionally call for ice, though I usually avoid it, because it waters down a smoothie. Sometimes that's what you want though. You may also want to freeze fruit juice, pureed fruit, or even coffee at some point. Chowhound recommends a silicone ice cube tray, because it's really easy to get out the cubes. Be sure the tray you select is BPA-free and dishwasher-safe. If you make a lot of smoothies with ice, get two trays, so you always have ice on hand.

Little food processor

Why is a food processor important? A food processor lets you make your own nut butter if you want, and it lets you grind down whole nuts, flaxseed, and oats into smaller, more blendable pieces. When you use pre-ground nuts, seeds, and oats, it's much easier on your blender's motor. This is the most expensive of the three extra pieces of smoothie equipment, but you don't have to spend an arm and a leg. You can get a good little processor for $40 or so. Whatever brand and model you choose, just make sure it's sturdy enough to make nut butter. That means it will definitely be up to chopping nuts, seeds, and grains.

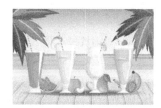

Chapter 3: Smoothie Shopping and Storing

You know the ingredients for a healthy smoothie and what kind of blender to get. What are some good shopping tips? How do you store the ingredients you get? In this chapter, I'll go through what to do before you go to the store, what to look for *at* the store, and how to store the fresh produce you buy.

Before the store

You've probably heard about meal planning at some point; maybe you even meal plan yourself. Even if you don't, I recommend at least planning out your week's worth of smoothies, so you always have the ingredients you need. A good thing about smoothies and the kinds of ingredients you buy is that you can switch them up, so you can decide on the fly that you want one with strawberries instead of raspberries. You aren't that tightly-tied to the smoothies you write down for the week.

Once you've chosen your smoothies, check to see if you have any of the ingredients already. A lot of these smoothies use ingredients you only use small amounts of at a time, and they last longer because they're frozen or they're spices, etc. When looking through your freezer, fridge, and pantry, you want to be well-stocked with ingredients that come up a lot in this book, like:

- Frozen berries (blueberries, strawberries, raspberries, etc.)
- Frozen cranberries/cranberry juice
- Frozen papaya
- Frozen cherries
- Frozen bananas
- Lemons
- Carrots
- Pineapple
- Wheatgrass powder
- Spirulina powder
- Fresh ginger
- Avocados
- Cucumbers
- Oranges/orange juice
- Oats
- Cinnamon
- Turmeric

- Vanilla extract
- Nut butter (almond butter, sunflower butter)
- Red grapes
- Pears
- Nut milk (almond/coconut)
- Greek yogurt
- Cottage cheese
- Tea (green/black)
- Dark leafy greens (especially spinach)
- Honey
- Chia seeds
- Flaxseed
- Nuts (e.g. pistachios, walnuts)

If you have most of these ingredients on hand at all times, you'll always be able to throw together a handful of the smoothies in this book. Of course, you won't be able to have *all* of these ingredients at all times, either because of space or season, so look to your smoothie guide and add what you don't have to your grocery list.

At the store

Once you're at the grocery store and looking for ingredients, what's the best type of produce to get? I always recommend organic, but that's not always possible based on what's available or your budget. If you want at least *some* of your fruits and veggies to be organic, take a look at the current year's "Dirty Dozen" list. This list lets you know what specific fruits and vegetables are the most affected by pesticides. Here's the top nine "dirtiest" for 2019, with #1 being the most concerning:

9. Pears
8. Cherries
7. Peaches
6. Grapes
5. Apples
4. Nectarines
3. Kale
2. Spinach
1. Strawberries

This means if you're buying strawberries, spinach, and kale, I highly recommend you buy organic. For other ingredients like nut milk, which can be pricey, I suggest you at least get a brand that's carcinogen-free. Look out specifically for "carrageenan," which is a substance made from red seaweed that serves as a thickener. It's natural, but carrageenan degrades in the liver and gastrointestinal tract. This can lead to inflammation. Bear in mind that organic nut milks can have carrageenan, so always look at the label to be sure. Silk and Califa Farms are common brands that don't contain carrageenan.

Last grocery store tip: fresh and frozen fruits and veggies have the same nutritional value. Buy frozen when you want to use the ingredient in the future, and fresh when you anticipate using it up pretty quickly, or there isn't a frozen alternative.

Storing ingredients

Not all fruits and vegetables should go in the fridge. Bananas, lemons, and limes should be kept in a cool, dry area. Mangos, plums, pears, and peaches can be kept at room temperature in a brown paper bag if they need to ripen, and then once they're ripe, stick them in the fridge to slow down the rotting process. Cantaloupe can be kept at room temperature, too, but it gets ripe very fast.

If you aren't using your apples within the week, store in the fridge. Carrots, berries, and most other fruit can also go in the fridge. For maximum freshness, store grapes, strawberries, cherries, and other berries in a plastic bag with tiny holes. This allows moisture to escape. Keep all fridge fruits and veggies in a crisper drawer.

Freezing produce

What about freezing fresh fruit and vegetables? With fruit, you want it to be in small enough pieces to blend easily. Berries are already small, so just wash and dry them well first, but bananas can be peeled and cut in half or chunks before you put them in a freezer bag and freeze. Fruit like mango, papaya, and strawberries can be sliced first, too. For the best results, make sure the fruit is really dry, and then put on a baking sheet lined with parchment paper. Arrange fruit in a single layer on the sheet, cover with plastic wrap, and then freeze till solid. The frozen fruit can then be taken off the parchment paper and put in freezer bags. They'll last 6-9 months with this method. If you just want to throw some ripe fruit in a bag and not bother with the parchment paper and baking sheet, that's fine, too. They just might end up with freezer burn at some point. If you're going to use the frozen fruit pretty soon, it's fine to just put it in a freezer bag right away.

What about dark leafy greens? You'll use your baking sheet again. Wash and dry leaves really well. Tear into smaller pieces and then lay out on a parchment-lined baking sheet. Freeze until solid, then quickly transfer to freezer bags. Greens frozen this way should last about 6 months.

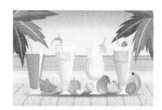

Chapter 4: Smoothie Do's and Don'ts

In this chapter, let's go over some useful tips for making the best healthy smoothies. There are certain things you should do, and things you should avoid. Smoothies, depending on their ingredients, can be healthy, not-so healthy, and even downright unhealthy. By reading the do's and don'ts, you can be sure to always make the healthiest smoothie possible. At the end of the chapter, I'll answer five frequently-asked questions about smoothies and cancer.

DO: Make green smoothies frequently

If you drink smoothies a lot, be sure you're balancing deliciously-sweet fruit smoothies with green ones. Dark leafy greens are packed with nutrients great for people wanting to prevent cancer and those going through cancer treatment. They are also usually lower in sugar than fruit smoothies.

DON'T: Go crazy with the added sweeteners

Especially in the United States, people are used to very sweet food. If you are new to homemade smoothies, you'll probably think they aren't sweet enough. You'll be tempted to add honey, agave, and maple syrup to make a smoothie taste sweeter, and while a little is okay, it's very easy to add too much. A healthy smoothie can quickly become dessert. We have some dessert smoothies in this book, but even those don't have a lot of added sweeteners.

Tip: If you're really concerned about sweeteners and want to avoid as many as often as you can, consider natural 0-calorie sweeteners like liquid stevia. It is hundreds of times sweeter than sugar, so you need very little. However, some people do experience side effects, like headaches, and sometimes stevia leaves a bitter aftertaste. If you're replacing a sweetener like honey in a smoothie, you'll want to use much less stevia. Start with just one drop and taste.

DO: Make breakfast smoothies the night before

In general, I recommend drinking a smoothie as soon as you make it, but for breakfast, making it the night before is a great idea if you are short on time in the morning. It will probably taste basically the same, and you're guaranteed a healthy and nourishing breakfast.

DON'T: Get a low-quality blender

Blenders are so important, I spent a whole chapter on them. In case you are still tempted to get the cheapest blender you can find, I'm reminding you how essential a good model is. A lot of these recipes use frozen ingredients, ice, and root vegetables like carrots, and a cheap, low-quality blender will not be able to handle these well, if at all. You might end up breaking your blender or making smoothies you don't like drinking. Get a good blender, and you'll be able to consistently make great smoothies.

DO: Use nut milks and yogurt for your smoothie base

Pretty much all the recipes in this book use nut milk, nonfat Greek yogurt, or both. Why not regular milk? Cow's milk has lots of sugar and has been linked to inflammation. A lot of cow's milk is also produced by animals given lots of hormones and other chemicals. Organic milk is better, so if you really want to use cow's milk in a smoothie for some reason, choose organic. You will pay more for the privilege, and taste-wise, I don't find it makes a huge difference. As for why you should use nonfat Greek yogurt, it's a great thickener and adds protein. Yogurt is also believed to have anti-inflammatory effects.

Frequently-Asked Questions

Hopefully, I've preemptively answered a lot of questions you might have about what ingredients to use in your smoothies and what to look for in a blender, but there might be more. Here are five frequently-asked questions and their answers:

What's the difference between making homemade juices with a juicer and smoothies?

You'll often see health blogs or experts talking about juices and smoothies. You can juice at home, with a juicer, just like you can make smoothies at home. However, juicers remove the pulp from the ingredients. You end up with strained juice in a glass and a weird plug of dry pulp in another part of the machine. With smoothies, there is no straining. Everything gets blended in one jug.

Are smoothies healthier than juices?

It depends on what you're looking for. With juices, the fiber is extracted with all the pulp. This makes juices easier to digest, but if you want the benefits of fiber, you'll be missing out. Smoothies keep all the fiber, so you're drinking whole veggies and fruit. Smoothies are better as meal replacements because they actually make you feel full, while juices don't. There's no evidence that shows juices are healthier than whole fruits and vegetables, and considering that juicing takes more fruit and veggies to get the same amount of a smoothie, and cleaning a juicer is more work, I think smoothies are a better choice for cancer-prevention and cancer treatment.

Why can't I just buy smoothies instead of making them?

Smoothies are pretty easy to make, but not as easy as simply buying a smoothie from the store or a smoothie shop. Why should you make them yourself? There are two big reasons. First off, you're in control of the ingredients when you blend your own drinks. Bottled smoothies often contain a *lot* of sugar and preservatives. They simply aren't that healthy. You also can't choose the specific cancer-preventing ingredients you want, or the ingredients that can help with cancer treatment. You're boxed into what the company chooses to produce. Bottled smoothies and smoothies from a shop are also pretty expensive. You'll pay more for 12-ounces of commercial smoothie than for the ingredients of a 12-ounce homemade smoothie. Does this mean you can *never* go out and buy a smoothie? Of course not. However, if you want the most benefits possible for an affordable price, depend on homemade smoothies.

Can healthy smoothies prevent cancer?

This is a book about smoothies that can help reduce your risk for cancer and help during cancer treatment, but I want to be clear about health claims. There is no guarantee against cancer. I also want to be clear that anything I say in this book should not replace professional medical advice. You could make all the cancer-preventing smoothies in this book on a regular basis, and still be diagnosed with cancer one day. You could be diagnosed with cancer, and make all the smoothies with ingredients that can inhibit the spread of cancer, and not see any improvements.

I obviously hope that doesn't happen, for so many reasons, but the harsh reality is that healthy smoothies are not a magic cure-all. However, these smoothies can be part of a healthy diet, and studies show that a healthy and balanced diet does indeed lower a person's risk for cancer. A healthy diet can also help heal damage from cancer treatment, and give the body a fighting chance against disease.

Besides making healthy smoothies, what can I do to lower my risk for cancer?

I've said smoothies can be part of a healthy lifestyle, so what else can you do to protect yourself against cancer? A healthy diet is a big one, so eat lots of vegetables, good proteins, and reduce your consumption of processed and refined foods. Exercise is also important. Together, a healthy diet and exercise can help you stay at a healthy weight, since obesity is linked to a variety of cancers. Some other tips: limit your alcohol intake and don't use tobacco products. Lastly, get regular cancer screening tests, so any red flags can be caught as early as possible.

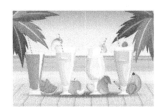

Chapter 5: Fruity Smoothies (For Cancer Prevention)

The smoothies in this section have been specifically selected for their cancer-preventing fruity ingredients, like apples, red grapes, cranberries, and more. While many of them could be enjoyed during cancer treatment, some may contain ingredients that might counteract with drugs, so that's why I have a separate section just for smoothies during treatment. Fruit smoothies are a great choice for breakfast, though they can also serve as refreshing treats on hot summer days.

Raspberry-Grape Smoothie
Apple + Carrot Smoothie
Cran-Apple Smoothie (Cranberry + Apple)
Papaya-Coconut Smoothie
Blueberry-Banana Smoothie
Cherry-Berry Smoothie
Straw-Melon Smoothie (Strawberry + Watermelon)
Nectarine + Raspberry Chia Smoothie
Coconut-Blackberry Smoothie
Pear-Berry Smoothie (Pear + Blueberry)
Classic Mango Smoothie
Mango Smoothie (With Turmeric)
Pistachio-Berry Smoothie

Raspberry-Grape Smoothie

Serves: 1

Red grapes are naturally quite sweet, so you don't need any added sugar in this smoothie, unless you count a handful of raspberries, which are packed with cancer-preventing antioxidants. You can use fresh or frozen. The yogurt thickens the smoothie and adds protein.

Ingredients:
 ¼ cup water
 ½ cup plain nonfat Greek yogurt
 1 cup red seedless grapes
 ½ cup fresh or frozen raspberries
 ½ small frozen banana

Directions:
Pour water into your blender. Add yogurt, then grapes and raspberries. Top with banana. Blend until smooth.

Nutritional Info:
 Total calories: 246
 Carbs: 56.4
 Fat: 0.6
 Fiber: 7.8
 Protein: 8.3

Apple + Carrot Smoothie

Serves: 1

This gorgeously-colorful smoothie is free from any refined sugars and gets its sweetness naturally from the carrot, apple, and banana. Nutritionally, it's full of antioxidants and fiber. It's a great smoothie for breakfast, with the sweet-spiciness of cinnamon alerting your senses for the day.

Ingredients:

1 cup unsweetened almond milk
2 chopped carrots
1 chopped apple
1 frozen banana
1 teaspoon grated ginger
Pinch of cinnamon

Directions:

Pour almond milk into your blender, followed by carrots, apple, and bananas. Blend until smooth, then stir in the ginger and cinnamon with a spoon. If it's too thick for your liking, thin with water.

Nutritional Info:

Total calories: 296
Carbs: 67.9
Fat: 4.2
Fiber: 12
Protein: 3.7

Cran-Apple Smoothie (Cranberry + Apple)

Serves: 1

Sweet and tart, this smoothie is a great choice for breakfast. Three of its five ingredients are known to fight cancer, as well as boost the immune system. If you find the smoothie too tart, use a sweeter type of apple or add a little more honey.

Ingredients:
    ½ cup unsweetened almond milk
    ½ teaspoon honey
    ½ chopped apple
    ½ cup frozen cranberries
    ½ small frozen banana

Directions:

Pour almond milk into your blender, then add honey, apple, and finish with frozen banana and cranberries. Blend until smooth.

Nutritional Info:
    Total calories: 149
    Carbs: 33.3
    Fat: 2.1
    Fiber: 5.5
    Protein: 1.4

Papaya-Coconut Smoothie

Serves: 1

Tropical and lightly-sweetened, this smoothie uses both papaya fruit and papaya leaf extract, which you can buy from Amazon. The extract doesn't have any flavor, so you could technically add it to any of the smoothies in this book; it just makes sense to add it here. Some brands aren't cheap, but you use so little at a time, it will last a while. Also in this smoothie is coconut milk, yogurt, a banana, and ice, which helps thicken the drink. You can enjoy this for breakfast or as a snack.

Ingredients:
½ cup unsweetened coconut milk (from a carton)
1 serving papaya leaf extract
¼ cup nonfat Greek yogurt
½ peeled and sliced banana
¼ cup large papaya
½ cup ice

Tip: *If you can't find papaya, substitute with cantaloupe, which has a similar flavor. If you want to stay in the tropics, use mango, though the flavor is distinct from papaya.*

Directions:
Pour coconut milk into your blender and add papaya leaf extract. Follow with yogurt, banana and papaya, and top with ice. Blend until smooth.

Nutritional Info:
Total calories: 201
Carbs: 25.9
Fat: 9.5
Fiber: 2.7
Protein: 5.3

Blueberry-Banana Smoothie

Serves: 1

This simple blueberry smoothie is great for breakfast or snacks on a warm day. The Greek yogurt gives the smoothie some protein and thickness, while the banana adds sweetness. You can use either fresh or frozen blueberries.

Ingredients:

1 cup water
½ cup nonfat Greek yogurt
1 cup fresh or frozen blueberries
1 frozen banana

Directions:

Pour water into your blender, followed by yogurt and blueberries. Top with frozen banana. Blend until smooth.

Nutritional Info:

Total calories: 253
Carbs: 58.5
Fat: .9
Fiber: 8.1
Protein: 8.4

Cherry-Berry Smoothie

Serves: 1

This vibrantly-colored smoothie is packed with antioxidants thanks to blueberries, cherries, and raspberries. It's a little on the tart side, so add a little honey if you find it too sour. You can use fresh or frozen fruit, though frozen fruit will probably result in a slightly thicker smoothie.

Ingredients:
½ cup unsweetened almond milk
½ teaspoon honey (optional)
1 cup blueberries
1 cup pitted sour cherries
½ cup raspberries

Directions:
Pour milk into your blender. Add honey if using, and then all the berries. Blend until smooth.

Nutritional Info (w/ honey):
Total calories: 215
Carbs: 50.2
Fat: 2.7
Fiber: 8.5
Protein: 2.8

Straw-Melon Smoothie (Strawberry + Watermelon)

Serves: 1

This simple 3-ingredient smoothie is big on flavor. Strawberries and watermelon combine into a deliciously-sweet and refreshing beverage that you'll want to sip all summer long. Because both fruits are naturally sweet, you don't need any additional sweeteners.

Ingredients:

- ½ cup unsweetened almond milk
- ½ cup sliced strawberries
- 1 cup chopped seedless watermelon

Directions:

Pour milk into your blender. Add strawberries and watermelon, then blend until smooth.

Nutritional Info:

- Total calories: 89
- Carbs: 18
- Fat: 2.2
- Fiber: 2.5
- Protein: 1.9

Nectarine + Raspberry Chia Smoothie

Serves: 1

Nectarines are a favorite summer fruit, and their sweetness is highlighted by the slight tartness of raspberries. For extra nutrients like fiber and protein, add just a tablespoon of chia seeds.

Ingredients:

  1 cup unsweetened almond milk
  1 cup sliced nectarines
  ½ cup fresh or frozen raspberries
  1 tablespoon of chia seeds

Directions:

Pour milk into your blender. Add nectarines, raspberries, and chia seeds. Blend until smooth.

Nutritional Info:

  Total calories: 191
  Carbs: 29.9
  Fat: 9.3
  Fiber: 12.4
  Protein: 6.2

Coconut-Blackberry Smoothie

Serves: 1

Blackberries are kind of the black sheep of the berry family. This is unfortunate, because they are not only full of antioxidants, they are delicious. Slightly tart, with a sweet aftertaste, these berries are a great addition to smoothies like this one. The tartness is mellowed out by a banana for sweetness and coconut milk. You're actually going to use coconut cream in addition to milk from a carton, because it's creamier.

Ingredients:

¾ cup unsweetened coconut milk (from a carton)
1 tablespoon coconut cream
½ cup blackberries
½ frozen banana

Directions:

Pour coconut milk and cream into your blender, then add blackberries and banana. Blend until smooth.

Nutritional Info:

Total calories: 152
Carbs: 22.7
Fat: 7.5
Fiber: 6.4
Protein: 2

Pear-Berry Smoothie (Pear + Blueberry)

Serves: 1

Antioxidant-rich blueberries and pears have different growing seasons, which is why I recommend using frozen blueberries for this recipe. Despite the difference in their harvests, pears and blueberries go very well together since they are both sweet, with the blueberry's slight tanginess complimenting a ripe pear's sugary qualities. If you think the smoothie will be sweet enough, leave out the honey.

Ingredients:

⅔ cup unsweetened coconut milk (from a carton)

1 teaspoon honey

1 cup sliced pears

½ cup frozen blueberries

Directions:

Pour coconut milk into your blender, then add honey and pears. Top with frozen blueberries. Blend until smooth.

Nutritional Info:

Total calories: 186

Carbs: 42.1

Fat: 3.2

Fiber: 7.4

Protein: 1.2

Classic Mango Smoothie

Serves: 1

Mango, which has been shown to help prevent certain cancers, is a perfect tropical fruit. It's not too sweet and it enhances the coconut and banana in this smoothie. Nonfat Greek yogurt adds texture and nutrients like protein, while the optional honey sweetens the overall flavor.

Ingredients:

½ cup unsweetened coconut milk (from a carton)
1 teaspoon honey (optional)
½ cup plain nonfat Greek yogurt
½ fresh banana
1 cup frozen mango

Directions:

Add milk and honey to your blender, and then yogurt. Finish with the fresh banana and frozen mango. Blend until smooth.

Nutritional Info (w/ honey):

Total calories: 283
Carbs: 56.6
Fat: 4.8
Fiber: 6.7
Protein: 8

Mango Smoothie (With Turmeric)

Serves: 1

This anti-inflammatory fruit smoothie includes turmeric, a citrusy, bitter spice commonly used in Ayurvedic healing. The strong flavor of the spice is mellowed by honey, sweet mango, and a banana. You can use fresh or frozen mango.

Ingredients:
  1 cup unsweetened almond milk
  1 teaspoon honey
  1 teaspoon ground turmeric
  ½ cup fresh or frozen mango
  1 small frozen banana

Directions
Pour milk and honey into your blender. Add turmeric, mango, and banana. Blend until smooth.

Nutritional Info:
  Total calories: 208
  Carbs: 44.6
  Fat: 4.4
  Fiber: 5.4
  Protein: 3

Pistachio-Berry Smoothie

Serves: 1

As a tree nut, pistachios are full of anti-cancer nutrients and antioxidants, so they're a great addition to a smoothie. They're also very flavorful and turn a regular fruit smoothie into something a bit more interesting. We're using three kinds of berries in this recipe, but you can use whatever berries you have on hand.

Ingredients:

½ cup unsweetened almond milk
¼ cup strawberries
¼ cup blueberries
¾ cup raspberries
2 tablespoons shelled pistachios

Directions:

Pour milk into your blender. Add berries, and then top with shelled pistachios. Blend until smooth.

Nutritional Info:

Total calories: 140
Carbs: 22
Fat: 6.1
Fiber: 8.9
Protein: 3.6

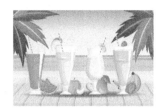

Chapter 6: Green Smoothies (Cancer Prevention + During Treatment)

Green smoothies often get a bad rap. A lot of people find they are too grassy or vegetal, and long for the sweetness of a fruity smoothie. They're also often too chunky and not blended properly, with lots of green bits floating around. However, when done right, green smoothies have more complex flavors, with more health benefits to boot.

While green smoothies are rarely as sweet as fruit ones, the more you drink them, the more you'll adjust to the sweetness level. It's like when you stop eating candy and then bite into a fresh strawberry, you are shocked at how sweet something natural is. This section is for smoothies made with greenies like spinach, kale, wheatgrass, avocados, and more. Unless otherwise stated, they can be made either for cancer prevention and during treatment, if you so desire.

Cucumber-Orange Smoothie (With Kale + Parsley)
Green-Applesauce Smoothie
Green Avocado-Banana Smoothie
Blueberry-Kale Smoothie
Berryful Green Smoothie
Gingery-Green Smoothie
Citrus Wheatgrass Smoothie
Beet-Green Pineapple Smoothie
Spirulina-Blackberry Smoothie
Banana-Coconut Smoothie (With Spirulina)
Green Pear Smoothie
Spinach Strawberry-Grape Smoothie
Cranberry-Pear Smoothie (With Swiss Chard)
Pistachio Green Smoothie

Cucumber-Orange Smoothie (With Kale + Parsley)

Serves: 1

Citrusy and refreshing, this is a great smoothie for hot days when you need to get in your veggies. The parsley (which shouldn't be eaten with cancer treatment drugs) adds cancer-preventing nutrients and fresh flavor, while the potentially-bitter kale is sweetened by banana and orange juice. The cucumber doesn't add much for flavor, but it's very hydrating.

Ingredients:

½ cup 100% orange juice
½ cup cucumber
½ cup parsley
¾ cup kale leaves
½ small frozen banana

Directions:

Pour orange juice into your blender. Add cucumber, parsley, and kale. Top with frozen banana. Blend until smooth.

Nutritional Info:

Total calories: 128
Carbs: 35
Fat: 0
Fiber: 2
Protein: 6

Green-Applesauce Smoothie

Serves: 1

Sweetened by applesauce and pineapple, this is a great green smoothie if you don't really like green smoothies. Kale and spinach are both very nutrient-rich, but you can't really taste them. If you don't have pineapple on hand, you can substitute pretty much any kind of fruit.

Ingredients:

    ½ cup coconut water
    ¼ cup unsweetened applesauce
    1 cup kale
    1 cup spinach
    ½ cup pineapple

Directions:

Pour coconut water and applesauce in your blender. Add kale and spinach, then fresh or frozen pineapple on top. Blend until smooth.

Nutritional Info:

    Total calories: 132
    Carbs: 32.3
    Fat: .3
    Fiber: 3.5
    Protein: 3.4

Green Avocado-Banana Smoothie

Serves: 1

This silky-smooth smoothie is simple and delicious. There's flaxseed for nutrients like fiber and protein, and spinach for antioxidants. The avocado and banana both add richness and thickness, so if you find the smoothie *too* thick, thin with a little water.

Ingredients:
½ cup unsweetened almond milk
1 tablespoon ground flaxseed
1 cup spinach
½ avocado
½ frozen banana

Directions:
Pour almond milk in your blender. Add flaxseed, spinach, avocado, and frozen banana. Blend until smooth.

Nutritional Info:
Total calories: 261
Carbs: 25
Fat: 17.6
Fiber: 10.5
Protein: 5

Blueberry-Kale Smoothie

Serves: 1

Kale and blueberries are often found together in summer salads, so they make sense together in a smoothie. Great for breakfast, this smoothie also has almond milk, Greek yogurt, and chia seeds for all the nutrients you need to start the day right.

Ingredients:
¾ cup unsweetened almond milk
½ cup nonfat Greek yogurt
1 cup kale
1 tablespoon of chia seeds
½ cup fresh or frozen blueberries

Directions:
Pour almond milk and Greek yogurt into your blender. Add kale, chia seeds, and fresh or frozen blueberries. Blend until smooth.

Nutritional Info:
Total calories: 228
Carbs: 35.5
Fat: 7.9
Fiber: 10
Protein: 12.3

Berryful Green Smoothie

Serves: 1

Another good recipe if you're just getting into green smoothies, this one blends strawberries, raspberries, a banana, and coconut milk with spinach. You'll barely notice the greens with the fruity flavors, but you'll get all the spinach's cancer-preventing antioxidants.

Ingredients:

1 cup unsweetened coconut milk (from a carton)
2 cups spinach
½ cup strawberries
½ cup raspberries
1 small frozen banana

Directions:

Pour coconut milk into your blender. Add spinach, berries, and banana. Blend until smooth.

Nutritional Info:

Total calories: 204
Carbs: 40.1
Fat: 5.2
Fiber: 10.4
Protein: 4

Gingery-Green Smoothie

Serves: 1

Packed with antioxidants and anti-inflammatory ingredients, this smoothie is a good choice for building up the immune system and healing during cancer treatment. Ginger helps with nausea, while turmeric may help slow down cancer growth. The "green" in the recipe comes from spinach.

Ingredients:

1 cup coconut water
1 cup spinach
Handful of fresh parsley
1-inch thumb of grated ginger
1 teaspoon turmeric
½ frozen banana

Directions:

Pour water into your blender. Add spinach, parsley, ginger, and turmeric. Top with frozen banana. Blend until smooth.

Nutritional Info:

Total calories: 97
Carbs: 24
Fat: 0
Fiber: 2.2
Protein: 2

Citrus Wheatgrass Smoothie

Serves: 1

Wheatgrass can be a polarizing ingredient. It tastes like, well, grass, but in this smoothie, orange juice helps neutralize those stronger flavors. A banana helps, too, and sweetens the smoothie. For some extra protein and fiber, add a tablespoon of chia seeds.

Ingredients:

1 cup of orange juice
¼ teaspoon wheatgrass powder
1 tablespoon of chia seeds
½ frozen banana

Tip: Wheatgrass powder

You can buy or even grow wheatgrass, but many find it more convenient to get wheatgrass powder. You want a really good brand, preferably organic, to get the most health benefits without additives. Garden of Life is a good brand that blends well.

Directions:

Pour orange juice into your blender. Add wheatgrass powder, chia seeds, and banana. Blend until smooth.

Nutritional Info:

Total calories: 223
Carbs: 44
Fat: 4
Fiber: 7
Protein: 5

Beet-Green Pineapple Smoothie

Serves: 1

Beet greens aren't used as often as they should be for smoothies. When you buy beets, save the greens for this smoothie. They are full of vitamin C, A, iron, calcium, and more. They taste like a slightly-sweeter Swiss chard, but you'll probably taste more of the pineapple and banana in this smoothie.

Ingredients:

½ cup coconut water
2 cups beet greens
1 cup cucumber
½ cup pineapple
1 small frozen banana

Directions:

Pour water into your blender. Add beet greens, cucumber, and fresh or frozen pineapple. Finish off with banana. Blend until smooth.

Nutritional Info:

Total calories: 229
Carbs: 57
Fat: 0
Fiber: 8
Protein: 5

Spirulina-Blackberry Smoothie

Serves: 1

Spirulina is a popular smoothie ingredient these days and after glancing at the health benefits, it's easy to see why. The blue-green algae is packed with nutrients, and very easy to add in power form. In this recipe, you blend coconut milk with spinach, spirulina, blackberries, and a frozen banana into a beautiful dark blue-green smoothie.

Ingredients:

    1 cup unsweetened coconut milk (from a carton)
    1 cup spinach
    ½ teaspoon organic spirulina
    ½ cup blackberries
    1 frozen banana

Tip: Spirulina

Spirulina is blue-green algae, and has a mild salty taste, like the ocean. Most importantly, it's rich in lots of antioxidants, vitamins, and minerals. It's best to buy organic spirulina powder from a brand like Triquetra or Micro Ingredients.

Directions:

Pour coconut milk into your blender. Add spinach, spirulina, blackberries, and banana. Blend until smooth.

Nutritional Info:

    Total calories: 200
    Carbs: 37.5
    Fat: 4.9
    Fiber: 8.6
    Protein: 5.2

Banana-Coconut Smoothie (With Spirulina)

Serves: 1

The goal of this smoothie is to hide the spirulina powder. We're not going to pretend that everyone loves the flavor of spirulina, or even likes it. In this smoothie, we're using ingredients to mask it, like coconut milk and coconut cream, cinnamon, honey, and banana.

Ingredients:
- 1 cup unsweetened coconut milk (from a carton)
- 1 tablespoon honey
- 1 tablespoon coconut cream
- ½ teaspoon cinnamon
- ½ teaspoon spirulina powder
- 1 frozen banana

Directions:
Pour coconut milk, honey, and coconut cream into your blender. Add cinnamon, spirulina powder, and frozen banana. Blend until smooth.

Nutritional Info:
- Total calories: 285
- Carbs: 56.6
- Fat: 7.6
- Fiber: 4.2
- Protein: 2.2

Green Pear Smoothie

Serves: 1

Pears have a naturally sugary-vanilla flavor, which is great for green smoothies. The coconut milk, banana, and touch of honey in this recipe also help balance out the potentially bitter spinach. If you aren't a fan of green smoothies usually, but really want the anti-cancer benefits, try this smoothie.

Ingredients:
⅔ cup unsweetened coconut milk (from a carton)
1 teaspoon honey
1 cup spinach
1 sliced pear
1 frozen banana

Directions:
Pour milk into your blender. Add honey, spinach, pear, and frozen banana. Blend until smooth.

Nutritional Info:
Total calories: 259
Carbs: 57
Fat: 4.7
Fiber: 9.1
Protein: 2.7

Spinach Strawberry-Grape Smoothie

Serves: 1

Strawberries and grapes are a deliciously-sweet pairing, and a great fruity compliment to spinach. You can use fresh or frozen strawberries, but frozen ones do add a frosty thickness to the smoothie that we really like.

Ingredients:

  1 cup unsweetened almond milk
  1 cup spinach
  ½ cup red grapes
  1 cup frozen strawberries

Directions:

Pour milk into your blender. Add spinach, red grapes, and frozen strawberries. Blend until smooth.

Nutritional Info:

  Total calories: 148
  Carbs: 28.5
  Fat: 4.1
  Fiber: 5.1
  Protein: 3.4

Cranberry-Pear Smoothie (With Swiss Chard)

***Serves:** 1*

With a similar flavor to spinach, Swiss chard is a great addition to a smoothie. It's very easily blended, thanks to tender leaves, and it's earthy, slightly bitter flavor goes well with sweet pears and tart cranberries.

Ingredients:

    1 cup unsweetened coconut milk (from a carton)
    1 generous handful of Swiss chard
    1 sliced pear
    1 cup frozen cranberries

Directions:

Pour coconut milk into your blender. Add Swiss chard and pear. Top with frozen cranberries.

Nutritional Info:

    Total calories: 162
    Carbs: 29.5
    Fat: 4.8
    Fiber: 7.9
    Protein: 1.2

Pistachio Green Smoothie

Serves: 1

This green smoothie gets a sweet nuttiness from pistachios, which are full of cancer-fighting antioxidants, fiber, and protein. Dark leafy greens boost the nutrition even more, and you can use whatever kind you have on hand. Ginger and honey add spice and sweetness, while a creamy avocado thickens the whole smoothie.

Ingredients:

> 1 cup unsweetened coconut milk (from a carton)
> 1 teaspoon honey
> 1 cup dark leafy green (your choice)
> ½ cup shelled pistachios
> ½ teaspoon fresh grated ginger
> ½ avocado

Directions:

Pour coconut milk and honey into your blender. Add the leafy green of your choice, then nuts and ginger. Top with avocado. Blend until smooth.

Nutritional Info:

> Total calories: 361
> Carbs: 22.2
> Fat: 30.8
> Fiber: 10
> Protein: 5.9

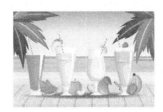

Chapter 7: Symptom Smoothies (During Treatment)

The smoothies in this section are all about treating the symptoms and side effects of cancer treatment. Your body goes through a lot during this time, and your immune system takes a big hit. A smoothie should contain ingredients known for their immune-boosting power. As a result of treatment and a weaker immune system, symptoms like loss of appetite, heartburn, nausea, and tasting metal are common. Many of the smoothies will be geared towards those problems.

Carrot-Ginger Smoothie with Turmeric
Pineapple-Ginger Smoothie
Classic Strawberry-Banana Smoothie (With a Twist)
Berry Lemonade Smoothie
Nutty-Nana Smoothie
Blueberry-Kiwi Chia Smoothie
Cantaloupe-Applesauce Smoothie
Prune-Raspberry Smoothie
Simple Orange Smoothie
Watermelon-Lime Smoothie
Lemony Ginger-Peach Smoothie
Apple-Pear Smoothie
Cranberry-Orange Smoothie
Cucumber-Apple Smoothie

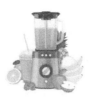

Carrot-Ginger Smoothie with Turmeric

Serves: 1

Turmeric is a known antioxidant and helps boost the immune system, which is important during treatment. This smoothie also has fresh ginger, which can help ease the nausea common during cancer treatment. Instead of whole carrots, we're using carrot juice, so the smoothie blends easier. You can get carrot juice from brands like Bolthouse Farms and Barsotti. A banana adds much-needed sweetness, since turmeric has a bitter flavor. If you don't like the taste of turmeric, you can add a little honey or agave to the smoothie to mask it a bit more.

Ingredients:
½ cup unsweetened almond milk
¼ cup organic carrot juice
¼ tablespoon grated ginger
¼ teaspoon ground turmeric
1 frozen banana

Directions:
Pour almond milk and carrot juice into your blender. Add grated ginger, turmeric, and frozen banana on top. Blend until smooth.

Nutritional Info:
Total calories: 138
Carbs: 31
Fat: 2.2
Fiber: 4.4
Protein: 2.1

Pineapple-Ginger Smoothie

Serves: 1

Tropical sweetness gets a little spicy kick from ginger in this smoothie. Pineapple is full of antioxidants and vitamins, and may boost the immune system. Ginger may also strengthen your immune system, and provide relief from nausea. Both ingredients combine in a delicious, health-promoting drink good for people recovering from cancer treatment.

Ingredients:
    1 cup water
    1 cup pineapple
    1-inch thumb of grated ginger
    ½ frozen banana

Directions:
Pour water into your blender, then add pineapple, ginger, and banana. Blend until smooth.

Nutritional Info:
    Total calories: 135
    Carbs: 35.1
    Fat: 0.4
    Fiber: 3.8
    Protein: 1.5

Classic Strawberry-Banana Smoothie (With a Twist)

Serves: 1

Strawberry and banana is a classic smoothie flavor combination. In this recipe, however, we add a little twist: ginger. It helps spice up the sweetness of the smoothie a little bit, and can help with nausea. You can use fresh strawberries instead of frozen if you want, though the drink might not be as thick.

Ingredients:

½ cup unsweetened almond milk
½-inch thumb of grated ginger
1 cup frozen strawberries
1 frozen banana

Directions:

Add milk, ginger, strawberries, and banana to your blender. Blend until smooth.

Nutritional Info:

Total calories: 171
Carbs: 39
Fat: 2.6
Fiber: 6.5
Protein: 2.8

Berry Lemonade Smoothie

Serves: 1

Perfect for summer, this lemonade smoothie is infused with all sorts of berries. If you prefer one berry over another, you can just use your favorite to make a strawberry-lemonade or raspberry-lemonade smoothie. Lemon is a really good palate cleanser for when you have "metal mouth."

Ingredients:
   ½ cup water
   2 tablespoons lemon juice
   ½ cup fresh or frozen mixed berries
   1 frozen banana

Directions:
Pour water and lemon juice in your blender. Add berries and banana. Blend until smooth.

Nutritional Info:
   Total calories: 152
   Carbs: 36.1
   Fat: 0.9
   Fiber: 5.7
   Protein: 2

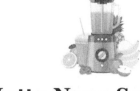

Nutty-Nana Smoothie

Serves: 1

This smoothie involves a teeny bit more prep than most smoothies. To make the nuts easily-blendable (and more digestible), you actually soak them overnight in a bowl of water. Other than that, besides the relatively normal freezing of a banana, this smoothie is just as easy to make as any other recipe. You end up with a drink that's sweet and nutty, and packed with nutrients great for the immune system, especially zinc.

Ingredients:
    1 cup unsweetened almond milk
    1 teaspoon honey
    1 tablespoon sunflower seeds
    1 tablespoon pumpkin seeds
    1 tablespoon ground flaxseed
    1 frozen banana
    Ice cubes

Tip: *The night before you plan on making your smoothie, put sunflower, pumpkin, and flaxseeds in a bowl and pour in enough water to cover them. Keep on the counter overnight. When you're going to make your smoothie, drain the seeds.*

Directions:
Pour almond milk into your blender, then add honey, soaked seeds, banana, and a few ice cubes. Blend until smooth.

Nutritional Info:
    Total calories: 267
    Carbs: 38.8
    Fat: 11.5
    Fiber: 6.6
    Protein: 6.3

Blueberry-Kiwi Chia Smoothie

Serves: 1

Blueberries and kiwis both have antioxidants, which are great for strengthening the immune system. Kiwis also taste a little like strawberries, so they add sweetness. That also makes it easy to swap out kiwis for strawberries, if necessary. For more nutrients known for helping the immune system, we've got chia seeds, which are a good source of zinc. Soak these for 10 minutes or so; they get a jelly-like texture instead of crunchy.

Ingredients:

¼ cup unsweetened coconut milk (from carton)
1 tablespoon of chia seeds
½ cup nonfat Greek yogurt
1 kiwi
½ cup frozen blueberries

Directions:

To soften chia seeds, cover with water and sit for 10 minutes. Once jelly-like, you're ready to make the rest of the smoothie. Pour coconut milk into your blender, then add chia seeds, yogurt, kiwi, and frozen blueberries. Blend until smooth.

Nutritional Info:

Total calories: 222
Carbs: 38.6
Fat: 6.8
Fiber: 10.8
Protein: 10.4

Cantaloupe-Applesauce Smoothie

Serves: 1

Cantaloupe, with its water content and low acidity, is a great fruit for relieving heartburn. Applesauce is also believed to help relieve symptoms because of alkalizing minerals like magnesium and potassium. Why are we adding turmeric, too? It has anti-inflammatory properties, and heartburn may be caused by inflammation. You only need a little.

Ingredients:
    ½ cup almond milk
    ½ cup unsweetened organic applesauce
    ½ cup cantaloupe
    ½ teaspoon turmeric

Directions:
Add almond milk, applesauce, cantaloupe, and turmeric to your blender. Puree until smooth.

Nutritional Info:
    Total calories: 332
    Carbs: 20.5
    Fat: 28.9
    Fiber: 4.5
    Protein: 3.6

Prune-Raspberry Smoothie

Serves: 1

When going through treatment, people often become constipated. To tackle the issue naturally, make this three-ingredient smoothie that includes prune juice. Prunes are a well-known laxative and work gently and quickly. You can swap in any kind of berry you want, if you have them on hand, instead of raspberries.

Ingredients:

½ cup unsweetened almond milk
½ cup organic prune juice
¼ cup raspberries

Directions:

Pour almond milk and prune juice into your blender, then add fresh or frozen raspberries. Blend until smooth.

Nutritional Info:

Total calories: 126
Carbs: 26.2
Fat: 2
Fiber: 3.5
Protein: 1.4

Simple Orange Smoothie

Serves: 1

Low energy is one of the most common symptoms of cancer treatment. Your body is going through a lot. Fatigue is a natural result. To boost your energy levels, try this orange smoothie. Oranges contain lots of ingredients known to help battle tiredness, like vitamin C and potassium. Best of all, the energy is released gradually instead of all at once, so you don't have to worry about a crash.

Ingredients:
½ cup unsweetened almond milk
1 peeled and sectioned orange
½ frozen banana
Ice cubes

Directions:
Pour milk into your blender. Add the orange pieces and then frozen banana on top. Toss in a few ice cubes. Blend until smooth.

Nutritional Info:
Total calories: 159
Carbs: 36.1
Fat: 2.2
Fiber: 6.5
Protein: 2.9

Watermelon-Lime Smoothie

Serves: 1

Extremely refreshing and hydrating, this smoothie mixes sweet watermelon and strawberries with the sourness of lime juice. Coconut water, which is known for its hydrating properties, is a great addition since it keeps the smoothie lighter than if you used nut milk, but it's more interesting than just plain water. You end up with a drink that's great for recovery after illness from cancer treatment, and great for metal mouth.

Tip: Coconut water

Coconut water has been around forever, but entered the drink market fairly recently. It contains nutrients like potassium, sodium, and calcium. It also has antioxidants. What brands are best? You want one that's as "clean," as possible, meaning without additives like sugar. On Epicurious, they looked at 19 brands and liked Zola (described as having a vanilla malt-lemony flavor), Harmless Harvest (an organic coconut water with a natural sweetness), and Whole Foods 365 (found at Whole Foods grocery stores).

Ingredients:

   ½ cup coconut water
   ½ teaspoon lime juice
   1 cup cubed seedless watermelon
   4 frozen strawberries

Directions:

Pour coconut water and lime juice into a blender. Add watermelon and strawberries. Blend until smooth.

Nutritional Info:

   Total calories: 136
   Carbs: 34
   Fat: 0.6
   Fiber: 2.2
   Protein: 2.1

Lemony Ginger-Peach Smoothie

Serves: 1

Ginger and peach go really well together. Peaches, which are very sweet, compliment and mellow out the unique spiciness of ginger. Lemon adds a layer of fresh tartness, while honey helps cut through some of that sourness. All together, the smoothie is a great blend of sweet and sour flavors for when you're feeling under the weather, fatigued, and/or nauseated.

Ingredients:
    ¾ cup unsweetened almond milk
    Juice of ½ lemon
    ½ tablespoon honey
    ½ tablespoon grated ginger
    1 cup peaches

Directions:
Pour milk, lemon juice, and honey into your blender. Add ginger and fresh or frozen peaches. Blend until smooth.

Nutritional Info:
    Total calories: 127
    Carbs: 24.6
    Fat: 3.2
    Fiber: 3.2
    Protein: 2.4

Apple-Pear Smoothie

Serves: 1

This sweet smoothie uses a whole pear, which are good for digestion problems like nausea, constipation, and diarrhea. For the apple, you'll want a sweet one, so there's no need for any added sweetener. A banana helps add sweetness and thickness. Sip this when you're having tummy troubles and need something in your stomach.

Ingredients:

1 cup unsweetened almond milk
½ sweet apple (like Gala, Golden Delicious, or Honeycrisp)
1 pear
1 frozen banana

Directions:

Pour almond milk into your blender. Add apple, pear, and frozen banana. Blend until smooth.

Nutritional Info:

Total calories: 283
Carbs: 65.5
Fat: 4.3
Fiber: 11.1
Protein: 3.1

Cranberry-Orange Smoothie

Serves: 1

To boost your immune system, which is weakened during cancer treatment, cranberries and oranges are both good fruits. In this smoothie, tart cranberry juice combines with a sweet orange, bananas, and nonfat Greek yogurt. It's not too sweet, not too sour, but just right. There's also a good amount of protein!

Ingredients:
½ cup unsweetened cranberry juice
½ cup plain nonfat Greek yogurt
1 segmented orange
1 frozen banana

Directions:
Pour cranberry juice into your blender, then add nonfat Greek yogurt. Pop in the orange segments, and then top with the frozen banana. Blend until smooth.

Nutritional Info:
Total calories: 297
Carbs: 68.6
Fat: 0.6
Fiber: 9
Protein: 9.1

Cucumber-Apple Smoothie

Serves: 1

Refreshing and cooling, this smoothie contains lemon and apple, both ingredients that can help with chemotherapy-triggered heartburn. Cucumber can also help with heartburn, as well as with hydration. Add a pinch of cinnamon for flavor.

Ingredients:

1 cup unsweetened coconut milk (from a carton)
1 tablespoon lemon juice
½ sweet apple
½ cup chopped cucumber
Pinch of cinnamon

Directions:

Pour coconut milk and lemon juice into your blender. Add apple, cucumber, and cinnamon. Blend until smooth.

Nutritional Info:

Total calories: 114
Carbs: 19.6
Fat: 4.4
Fiber: 4
Protein: 0.8

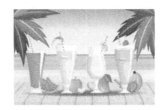

Chapter 8: Protein Smoothies (During Treatment)

During cancer treatment, doctors often recommend that patients eat more protein. This nutrient is essential for cell growth, cell repair, and a healthy immune system. If you aren't getting enough protein, your body will have trouble recovering. Lots of food is high in protein, but eating a steak might not be very appealing to a lot of people during treatment. Smoothies are a great way to add more protein to your diet, especially plant-based protein. The recipes in this section use protein-rich ingredients like oats, nut butters, and high-quality, plant-based protein powders. The smoothies without protein powder have less protein, but use more natural ingredients and tend to be lower calorie.

Tip: Protein powders

What kind of protein powder should you get? There's a lot of not-so-great brands out there full of chemicals and additives. I recommend plant-based proteins like pea or hemp. Orgain Organic, which has 21 grams of protein per serving, mixes organic pea protein, chia seeds, and organic brown rice protein. Aloha is another brand to consider. They use pea protein, organic hemp protein, and organic pumpkin seed protein. In terms of servings, we generally stick to two tablespoons, but you can add more if desired.

For the nutritional info, I calculated the information using Optimal Plant Proteins Protein Powder from Jarrow Formulas. Depending on what you use, the nutritional will be simply different.

Banana-Cinnamon Protein Smoothie

Peanut Butter-Banana Oatmeal Smoothie

Pineapple-Papaya Protein Smoothie

Berry Sunbutter Oatmeal Smoothie

Peanut Butter + J-Chia Seed Protein Smoothie

Cherry-Vanilla Smoothie (with Flaxseed)

Cranberry-Almond Butter Smoothie

Ruby-Red Berry-Beet Protein Smoothie

Peanut Butter-Sweet Potato Smoothie

Peachy-Cottage Cheese Smoothie

Nectarine-Walnut Smoothie

Banana-Cashew Smoothie

Mango Quinoa Smoothie

Berry Chickpea Protein Smoothie

Banana-Cinnamon Protein Smoothie

Serves: 1

A great smoothie for mornings, this banana-based recipe uses protein powder. A vanilla-flavored powder fits with the other ingredients. If you really love cinnamon, feel free to add more, but start with 1 teaspoon and taste.

Ingredients:
1 cup unsweetened almond milk
1 teaspoon cinnamon
2 tablespoons plant powder (vanilla-flavored)
1 frozen banana

Directions:
Add milk, cinnamon, and powder to your blender. Add frozen banana. Blend until smooth.

Nutritional Info:
Total calories: 301
Carbs: 40.8
Fat: 6.9
Fiber: 10.3
Protein: 23.4

Peanut Butter-Banana Oatmeal Smoothie

Serves: 1

Oats and peanut butter both contain protein, so this is a good way to enjoy breakfast in smoothie form. Cinnamon, which has antioxidants, and salt add flavor to the relatively simple drink, while a banana sweetens it up, so you don't need another honey or sugar. If you have another nut butter on hand and no peanut butter, just use that instead. The best peanut butters have very few ingredients. MaraNatha's creamy no-stir natural peanut butter has just two: peanuts and salt.

Ingredients:

    1 cup unsweetened almond milk
    ¼ cup rolled oats
    1 tablespoon smooth peanut butter
    ½ teaspoon cinnamon
    1 frozen banana
    Pinch of salt

Tip: *To make the smoothie easier to blend, pulse your oats through a food processor a few times before adding to blender.*

Directions:

Put milk, oats, and peanut butter in your blender. Add cinnamon, frozen banana, and a pinch of salt. Blend until smooth.

Nutritional Info:

    Total calories: 319
    Carbs: 46.9
    Fat: 13.3
    Fiber: 7.7
    Protein: 9

Pineapple-Papaya Protein Smoothie

Serves: 1

Fresh and tropical, this smoothie uses creamy almond butter for its protein. The nutty sweetness balances really well with the more acidic sweetness of the pineapple. The papaya, with its hydrating flavor and nutritional properties, is a great addition. If you don't have papaya, you can substitute with mango, and it will still taste delicious, though slightly different.

Ingredients:
    1 cup unsweetened coconut milk (from a carton)
    1 ½ tablespoons smooth almond butter
    ¾ cup pineapple
    ¾ cup papaya

Directions:
Add coconut milk, almond butter, pineapple, and papaya to your blender. Blend until smooth.

Nutritional Info:
    Total calories: 438
    Carbs: 37.5
    Fat: 30
    Fiber: 8.1
    Protein: 10.2

Berry Sunbutter Oatmeal Smoothie

Serves: 1

Sunflower seed butter is often underrated as a nut butter, but it's worth having a jar around, since sunflower seeds are a complete protein. They have other essential nutrients, too, like vitamin B, iron, and potassium. In this smoothie, you're basically enjoying a bowl of sunbutter oats with berries in liquid form.

Tip: Banana vs. avocado
You'll notice that instead of a banana, we're using an avocado, which adds thickness without the sugar content of a banana. If you're wondering about the taste, the berries and nut butter are strong enough to mask the very mild flavor difference. You can pretty easily replace a banana with ½ avocado or so in most smoothies.

Ingredients:
   1 cup unsweetened almond milk
   1 tablespoon sunflower seed butter
   ½ cup rolled oats
   ½ ripe avocado
   1 cup mixed berries

Directions:
Pour milk into your blender. Add sunflower seed butter, oats, avocado, and fresh or frozen berries. Blend until smooth.

Nutritional Info:
   Total calories: 573
   Carbs: 59.7
   Fat: 33.9
   Fiber: 16.9
   Protein: 12.4

Peanut Butter + J-Chia Seed Protein Smoothie

Serves: 1

Based on the classic peanut butter-and-jelly sandwich, this smoothie adds chia seeds for extra protein. Instead of jelly, use real strawberries, which are healthier. A frozen banana adds some more sweetness and texture.

Ingredients:

½ cup unsweetened almond milk
1 tablespoon smooth peanut butter
1 tablespoon of chia seeds
½ cup strawberries
½ frozen banana

Directions:

Pour almond milk into your blender. Add peanut butter, chia seeds, fresh or frozen strawberries, and frozen banana. Blend until smooth.

Nutritional Info:

Total calories: 248
Carbs: 29.1
Fat: 15.2
Fiber: 9.4
Protein: 8.6

Cherry-Vanilla Smoothie (with Flaxseed)

Serves: 1

Cherry and vanilla are a great combination. You can find them in Coca-Cola, but for a much healthier (and dare we say, tastier) version, make this smoothie. It uses almond milk and a little bit of vanilla extract for a boost of that fragrant flavor. The plant protein powder you use can also be vanilla-flavored. A banana and yogurt add thickness, while ground flaxseed gets that protein count higher. You can use sweet or sour cherries, though sour cherries have more health benefits.

Ingredients:
¼ cup unsweetened almond milk
¾ cup nonfat Greek yogurt
½ teaspoon vanilla extract
1 tablespoon ground flaxseed
2 tablespoons plant protein powder (vanilla-flavored)
1 cup frozen cherries
½ small frozen banana

Directions:
Pour milk, yogurt, and vanilla into your blender. Add flaxseed, plant protein powder, cherries, and banana. Blend until smooth.

Nutritional Info:
Total calories: 567
Carbs: 50.9
Fat: 23.7
Fiber: 11.2
Protein: 38.7

Cranberry-Almond Butter Smoothie

Serves: 1

The natural tartness of cranberries is mellowed by the rich nuttiness of almond butter in this lower-calorie protein smoothie. Chia seeds and yogurt add more protein and nutrients, while a banana replaces any refined sweeteners. If it's around the holidays, you might find fresh cranberries for a good price. Feel free to use them instead of frozen ones.

Ingredients:

¾ cup unsweetened coconut milk (from a carton)

½ cup plain nonfat Greek yogurt

1 tablespoon almond butter

1 tablespoon chia seeds

½ cup frozen cranberries

½ frozen banana

Directions:

Pour coconut milk into your blender. Add yogurt, almond butter, chia seeds, cranberries, and banana. Blend until smooth.

Nutritional Info:

Total calories: 337

Carbs: 39.5

Fat: 17.2

Fiber: 12.4

Protein: 13

Ruby-Red Berry-Beet Protein Smoothie

Serves: 1

This unusual smoothie looks beautiful - it's bright red or even pink. This is thanks to the strawberries, raspberries, and a beet. Why are we putting a beet in our smoothie? Beets are rich in antioxidants and nutrients like iron, potassium, fiber, and more. Raw beets taste earthy, even bitter, but those flavors are masked by the fruit, honey, and coconut milk. Beets also have a little protein, but to boost that, we're also blending in a plant protein powder and chia seeds.

Ingredients:

    1 cup unsweetened coconut milk (from a carton)
    1 teaspoon honey
    ½ cup strawberries
    ½ cup raspberries
    ½ tablespoon of chia seeds
    2 tablespoons plant protein powder
    1 small peeled and chopped beet

Directions:

Pour milk and honey into your blender. Add strawberries and raspberries (if fresh), and then chia seeds, protein powder, and chopped beet. If the berries are frozen, add them with the beet. Blend until smooth.

Nutritional Info:

    Total calories: 334
    Carbs: 43.6
    Fat: 10.3
    Fiber: 16
    Protein: 25.4

Peanut Butter-Sweet Potato Smoothie

Serves: 1

Peanut butter and sweet potato may seem like an odd combination, but it's actually not that strange. Sweet potatoes, normally a savory food, become sweeter when combined with the nutty goodness of peanut butter. You get both fiber and protein in this smoothie, thanks to the potato, peanut butter, flaxseed, and protein powder.

Ingredients:

1 cup unsweetened almond milk

1 tablespoon smooth peanut butter

1 tablespoon ground flaxseed

2 tablespoons plant protein powder

1 cup cooked sweet potato

½ frozen banana

Tip: *This recipe is best prepared when you already have a cooked sweet potato lying around. If you don't, you can buy canned cooked sweet potato. Just rinse off the sugary syrup first before adding to your smoothie.*

Directions:

Pour almond milk into your blender. Add peanut butter, ground flaxseed, protein powder, sweet potato, and banana. Blend until smooth.

Nutritional Info:

Total calories: 554

Carbs: 72

Fat: 72

Fiber: 17.1

Protein: 32

Peachy-Cottage Cheese Smoothie

Serves: 1

This tangy-sweet smoothie gets protein from two sources: chia seeds and cottage cheese. Peaches give the smoothie a beautiful pale-gold color and a burst of fruity sweetness perfect on a warm morning. For a little more sweetness to balance the tang of cottage cheese, add just a little honey. If you like the cottage cheese flavor, you can leave out the honey.

Ingredients:

½ cup unsweetened almond milk
½ tablespoon honey
½ cup cottage cheese
1 tablespoon of chia seeds
1 ½ cups frozen peaches

Directions:

Pour almond milk and honey into your blender. Add cottage cheese, chia seeds, and frozen peaches. Blend until smooth.

Nutritional Info:

Total calories: 300
Carbs: 40.7
Fat: 40.7
Fiber: 9
Protein: 21.2

Nectarine-Walnut Smoothie

Serves: 1

Walnuts, flaxseed, and nonfat Greek yogurt all add protein to this tasty smoothie. Nectarines, which taste like peaches, are a great counterpart to the intense nuttiness of walnuts and flaxseed. A frozen banana serves as a sweetener and thickener. You can use either fresh or frozen nectarines; you just add them at slightly-different times.

Ingredients:
¾ cup unsweetened almond milk
¾ cup nonfat Greek yogurt
1 nectarine
⅓ cup walnut pieces
1 tablespoon ground flaxseed
½ frozen banana

Directions:
Pour milk and yogurt into your blender. If using a fresh nectarine, add now, and then add walnuts and ground flaxseed. Add frozen banana last, and then blend until smooth. If your nectarine slices are frozen, add with the banana.

Nutritional Info:
Total calories: 684
Carbs: 43.4
Fat: 48.6
Fiber: 9.3
Protein: 24.3

Banana-Cashew Smoothie

Serves: 1

This is a very rich-tasting smoothie thanks to the fattiness of the cashews and the thickness the frozen banana adds. A bit of spicy cinnamon helps cut through that richness a little. Cashews have been shown to have anti-cancer properties, and provide some protein to this recipe. The main source of protein, however, comes from the plant protein powder.

Tip: *If you really want to "cashew" up this smoothie, replace almond milk with cashew milk from a brand like Silk.*

Ingredients:
    1 cup unsweetened almond milk
    ⅓ cup ground cashews
    ½ teaspoon cinnamon
    2 tablespoons plant protein powder
    1 frozen banana

Directions:
Pour 1 cup of milk into your blender. Before adding cashews, break them up a bit in your food processor. Add to the blender, along with cinnamon and protein powder. Top with frozen banana, then blend until smooth.

Nutritional Info:
    Total calories: 560
    Carbs: 54.8
    Fat: 28.1
    Fiber: 11.1
    Protein: 30.3

Mango Quinoa Smoothie

Serves: 1

Tropical with mango and pineapple, this smoothie uses quinoa as its protein. Quinoa is a great plant protein, and also a source for all nine essential amino acids. Nonfat Greek yogurt also adds protein, as well as creaminess. Since mango is pretty sweet, we're not adding any sweetener.

Ingredients:
½ cup unsweetened almond milk
¾ cup plain nonfat Greek yogurt
½ cup cooked quinoa
1 cup frozen mango

Directions:
Pour almond milk into your blender. Add nonfat Greek yogurt and cooked quinoa. Top with frozen mango. Blend until smooth.

Nutritional Info:
Total calories: 368
Carbs: 69.8
Fat: 4.3
Fiber: 8.8
Protein: 15.5

Berry Chickpea Protein Smoothie

Serves: 1

This normal berry smoothie has an unusual ingredient - chickpeas. Chickpeas are full of protein and have pretty much no flavor on their own, so they blend seamlessly with the other ingredients in this smoothie. You can substitute any other berry if you want.

Ingredients:
1 cup unsweetened almond milk
1 teaspoon honey
¼ cup cooked chickpeas
1 tablespoon of chia seeds
½ cup frozen raspberries

Directions:
Pour milk and honey into your blender. Add chickpeas, chia seeds, and frozen raspberries. Blend until smooth.

Nutritional Info:
Total calories: 219
Carbs: 32.3
Fat: 10
Fiber: 13.1
Protein: 8.4

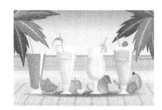

Chapter 9: Tea Smoothies (Cancer Prevention + During Treatment)

Tea is an underrated ingredient in smoothies. I wanted to devote a whole chapter to it because it's so versatile and pretty much all types have nutritional benefits of some kind, especially related to cancer prevention and treatment.

Green tea, while touted as the healthiest, is not the only brew you'll see in these recipes. There's also rich black tea, flavor, fragrant oolong tea and sweet, subtle white tea. When combined with classic smoothie ingredients like fruit, milk, and spices, you'll end up with unique, anti-cancer drinks for any time of day.

Raspberry-Green Tea Smoothie
Minty Peach-Green Tea Smoothie
Pineapple-Pistachio Green Tea Smoothie
Pear Chamomile Smoothie
Chamomile-Cherry Smoothie
Hibiscus-Raspberry Smoothie
Earl of Orange Smoothie
Coconut Chai-Chia Smoothie
Peach Oolong Smoothie
White Strawberry Smoothie
Peppermint Tea-Berry Smoothie
Lemon-Green Tea Protein Smoothie
Green Tea-Wheatgrass Smoothie

Raspberry-Green Tea Smoothie

Serves: 1

Refreshing and summery, this is the perfect smoothie for a hot day. The green tea and raspberries are packed with antioxidants, while the nonfat Greek yogurt adds protein and thickness. The whole thing is sweetened with honey. Another great thing about this recipe is that you can swap out raspberries with any other type of berry, or use a blend. Customize the fruit as you like.

Ingredients:

- 1 cup chilled brewed green tea
- 1 tablespoon honey
- ½ cup plain nonfat Greek yogurt
- 1 cup fresh or frozen raspberries
- ½ cup ice

Tip: How to brew green tea

There are a variety of green tea types with flavors ranging from grassy to toasty. They also brew at slightly-different water temperatures between 175-185 °F, so read the instructions on the tea you're using. For steeping, you should begin with 3 minutes and then taste. Avoid steeping the tea longer than 5 minutes, or it might become bitter. For best results, use purified or filtered water.

For this smoothie recipe, after straining the leaves or removing the bag, you want to cool to room temperature and then put in the fridge to chill.

Directions:

Pour chilled green tea into your blender. Add honey, yogurt, raspberries, and then finish off with ice. Blend until smooth.

Nutritional Info:

- Total calories: 193
- Carbs: 42.5
- Fat: 0.8
- Fiber: 9.5
- Protein: 7.5

Minty Peach-Green Tea Smoothie

Serves: 1

Peach tea is a Southern classic, and it gets a smoothie remix in this recipe. Use the same type of brewed tea from the recipe above, and swap out the raspberries for some fresh peaches. Some fresh mint really adds a lot, so don't skip the herb.

Ingredients:

1 cup chilled brewed green tea
½ tablespoon of honey
Small handful of fresh mint
1 cup sliced peaches

Directions:

Pour green tea into your blender. Add honey, mint, and peaches. Blend until smooth.

Nutritional Info:

Total calories: 91
Carbs: 22.7
Fat: 0.4
Fiber: 2.3
Protein: 1.4

Pineapple-Pistachio Green Tea Smoothie

Serves: 1

Blended with tropical pineapple, rich and sweet-nutty pistachios, and fresh green tea, this smoothie is a great choice for mornings when you need something light and bright. With antioxidants coming from the green tea, nuts, and pineapple, you'll be strengthening your body against all kinds of cancers.

Ingredients:

1 cup chilled green tea
1 teaspoon honey
2 tablespoons shelled pistachios
1 cup frozen pineapple

Directions:

Pour chilled green tea into your blender. Add honey, pistachios, and frozen pineapple. Blend until smooth.

Nutritional Info:

Total calories: 141
Carbs: 27.8
Fat: 3.5
Fiber: 3.8
Protein: 1.5

Pear Chamomile Smoothie

Serves: 1

Chamomile is a great tea for when you need sleep. Nutritionally, it's full of antioxidants that fight inflammation. It can also help soothe a troubled tummy, which pears can do as well. Together, with a little ginger, this is a great low-calorie smoothie for an evening when you're feeling ill from your cancer treatment and need good rest.

Tip: **Brewing chamomile**
You can use pretty hot water for chamomile, around 200-degrees. Steep for 5 minutes. Chill the tea before using in a smoothie.

Ingredients:

 1 cup chilled chamomile
 ½ teaspoon grated ginger
 ½ cup frozen pears

Directions:

Pour chilled chamomile into your blender. Add ginger and frozen pears. Blend until smooth.

Nutritional Info:

 Total calories: 47
 Carbs: 12.3
 Fat: 0.1
 Fiber: 2.5
 Protein: 0.3

Chamomile-Cherry Smoothie

Serves: 1

As you might know, chamomile tea is a great nighttime drink because it promotes relaxation. Tart cherries, with their melatonin content, are also a great snack at bedtime. Getting good sleep is essential to your overall health, so whether you're just trying to reduce your risk for cancer, or going through treatment, this rest-encouraging smoothie can help.

Ingredients:
    1 cup chilled chamomile tea
    1 teaspoon honey
    1 cup pitted fresh or frozen tart cherries

Directions:
Pour chilled tea into your blender and add honey. Top with fresh or frozen tart cherries, then blend.

Nutritional Info:
    Total calories: 81
    Carbs: 19.7
    Fat: 0
    Fiber: 2.1
    Protein: 1

Hibiscus-Raspberry Smoothie

Serves: 1

Hibiscus tea is a really refreshing choice for summer days. It's tart and sweet, a bit like cranberries, and goes really well with raspberries, which have a similar (but sweeter) flavor. You can substitute any other berry you want, or use a mix. What is hibiscus bringing to the table, nutritionally? It's rich in antioxidants and anthocyanins, which are known to reduce risk for chronic diseases like cancer.

Tip: **Hibiscus tea**

Hibiscus is becoming a popular tea flavor, so you can find bags of it from brands like Lipton. You can also find loose-leaf hibiscus from Amazon and other retailers that sell herbal tea. To brew with loose-leaf hibiscus tea, use about 2 tablespoons or so per cup, and steep in boiling water for 2-5 minutes. For cold-brew tea, steep 2 tablespoons with one cup of cold water for 8-12 hours.

Ingredients:

1 cup chilled hibiscus tea
¼ cup unsweetened almond milk
1 cup frozen raspberries

Directions:

Pour chilled tea into your blender and add milk. Add raspberries and blend until smooth.

Nutritional Info:

Total calories: 74
Carbs: 15.2
Fat: 1.7
Fiber: 8.3
Protein: 1.7

Earl of Orange Smoothie

Serves: 1

Earl grey is a classic English breakfast tea. It's a black tea, flavored with bergamot orange, which has a fragrant, citrusy flavor. In this smoothie, we're boosting that orange flavor with an actual orange for an energizing breakfast smoothie that contains antioxidants from the black tea, and nutrients like vitamin C and fiber.

Ingredients:
    1 cup of chilled Earl Grey tea
    ¼ cup unsweetened almond milk
    1 small orange

Directions:
Pour chilled tea into your blender and add milk. Top with orange segments, then blend until smooth.

Nutritional Info:
    Total calories: 55
    Carbs: 11.8
    Fat: 1
    Fiber: 2.6
    Protein: 1.2

Coconut Chai-Chia Smoothie

Serves: 1

Chai tea, which has a black tea base, is flavored with anti-cancer spices like cinnamon and ginger. The other spices in the tea like cardamom have also shown antioxidant properties. In this smoothie, coconut joins the party in the form of rich coconut cream, while nonfat Greek yogurt and chia seeds add nutrients like fiber and protein. To balance all that spice, a teaspoon of honey adds sweetness.

Ingredients:

    2 cups chilled chai tea

    1 teaspoon honey

    ¼ cup plain nonfat Greek yogurt

    1 tablespoon coconut cream

    1 tablespoon of chia seeds

Directions:

Pour chilled tea into your blender. Add honey, yogurt, coconut cream, and chia seeds. Blend until smooth.

Nutritional Info:

    Total calories: 180

    Carbs: 28.1

    Fat: 8.1

    Fiber: 5.8

    Protein: 6.2

Peach Oolong Smoothie

Serves: 1

Oolong, a traditional Chinese tea, has antioxidants, like all teas, and may have special qualities that fight breast cancer. In this smoothie, we're leaning into the tea's sweet side (it can have a range of tastes depending on the brand) with frozen peaches. Unsweetened almond milk serves as the blender.

Ingredients:

    1 cup chilled oolong tea
    ¼ cup unsweetened almond milk
    1 cup frozen peaches

Directions:

Pour tea and almond milk into your blender. Add frozen peaches. Blend until smooth.

Nutritional Info:

    Total calories: 69
    Carbs: 14.5
    Fat: 1.3
    Fiber: 2.6
    Protein: 1.7

White Strawberry Smoothie

Serves: 1

White tea is subtle and sweet, so even if you don't love tea, you'll love this smoothie. Strawberries bring out the tea's sweetness, though you can use any berry you want. For creaminess and some protein, add plain nonfat Greek yogurt, too.

Ingredients:
    1 cup chilled white tea
    ½ cup plain nonfat Greek yogurt
    1 cup frozen strawberries

Directions:
Pour tea into your blender and add yogurt. Top with frozen strawberries. Blend until smooth.

Nutritional Info:
    Total calories: 111
    Carbs: 21.6
    Fat: 0.4
    Fiber: 4.4
    Protein: 7

Peppermint Tea-Berry Smoothie

Serves: 1

Most smoothie recipes are for summer, but what about winter? Chilled peppermint tea (an herbal tea) is a great winter addition to smoothies because of how it wakes up your body. In this recipe, that crisp flavor mixes with raspberries for an antioxidant-rich kick that's perfect for mornings.

Ingredients:

1 cup chilled peppermint tea
½ tablespoon honey
1 cup of fresh or frozen raspberries

Tip: *You can buy peppermint tea in both loose leaf and bag form, but it's also very easy to make your own. Get some fresh peppermint leaves (or mint, they're basically the same) and steep for 5-10 minutes in boiling water. Strain the leaves, then chill for 3-4 hours before making your smoothie.*

Directions:

Pour chilled peppermint tea in your blender. Add honey first, and then fresh or frozen raspberries. Blend until smooth.

Nutritional Info:

Total calories: 96
Carbs: 23.3
Fat: 0.8
Fiber: 8
Protein: 1.5

Lemon-Green Tea Protein Smoothie

Serves: 1

This very simple smoothie takes a classic tea - green tea with honey and lemon - and makes it a protein-rich drink great for any time of the day. Both vanilla or unflavored protein powder work. A frozen banana thickens the smoothie and adds more sweetness, especially if you're used to adding more honey to your green tea.

Ingredients:

1 cup chilled green tea
1 teaspoon honey
1 ½ tablespoons fresh lemon juice
2 tablespoons plant protein powder (vanilla or unflavored)
½ frozen banana

Directions:

Pour green tea and honey in your blender. Add lemon juice, protein powder, and frozen banana. Blend until smooth.

Nutritional Info:

Total calories: 229
Carbs: 29.7
Fat: 3.4
Fiber: 6.6
Protein: 21.8

Green Tea-Wheatgrass Smoothie

Serves: 1

This very green smoothie uses green tea, spinach, and wheatgrass for an antioxidant-packed drink perfect for mornings. Lime juice and honey help balance out the grassy flavors, while half a frozen banana thickens up the whole thing.

Ingredients:
1 cup chilled brewed green tea
1 teaspoon honey
1 tablespoon lime juice
1 cup spinach
2 teaspoons wheatgrass powder
½ frozen banana

Directions:
Pour green tea, honey, and lime juice into your blender. Add spinach, wheatgrass, and frozen banana. Blend until smooth.

Nutritional Info:
Total calories: 119
Carbs: 26.1
Fat: 0.3
Fiber: 4.2
Protein: 3.6

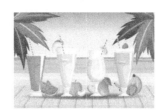

Chapter 10: Coffee Smoothies (Cancer Prevention)

Ah, coffee. It's the classic morning drink. If you're trying to replace your usual cup of Joe with a smoothie for health reasons, why not just combine the two beverages? In this section, I'm embracing coffee, which may have anti-cancer properties, and combining them with ingredients more associated closely with good health, like nonfat Greek yogurt, berries, and even spinach. If you're a sucker for peppermint coffee and pumpkin spice lattes, you'll find smoothies in here for you, too!

Note: **Making cold brew coffee**

You can find commercial cold brew coffee at pretty much any store, but how do you make your own concentrate, if that's something you want to do instead of just chilling regular coffee?

First, coarsely grind 8-ounces of good-quality beans. You want the consistency of raw sugar. Next, mix coffee with 2 quarts of water, and stir. Store in the fridge, covered, for 18-24 hours. Strain the concentrate, then mix with cold water using a 1:1 ratio. This diluted mix is what we're referring to in the recipes when we say "½ cup cold brew" or whatever recipe calls for.

The concentrate (undiluted) will last about 2 weeks in the fridge.

Vanilla Latte Smoothie
Cherry Latte Smoothie
A Berry Good Coffee Smoothie
Mocha Smoothie (With Flaxseed)
Shot In the Dark Smoothie
Green Coffee Smoothie
Hazelnut-Coffee Smoothie
Almond Butter Latte Smoothie
Mexican Coffee Smoothie
Pumpkin Spice Latte Smoothie
Peppermint Latte Smoothie
Vietnamese Coffee Smoothie (With Chia Seeds)
Almond Joy Coffee Smoothie

Vanilla Latte Smoothie

Serves: 1

A latte - coffee with milk - is a classic beverage. It gets "smoothie-fied" in this recipe with cold brew, almond milk, and nonfat Greek yogurt for some protein. If you like a stronger vanilla taste, use the full teaspoon (or more!) of pure extract if you want. For a really clean latte taste, you'll notice there's no banana in this recipe. For a sweetener, we're using honey.

Ingredients:
½ cup cold brew coffee
¾ cup unsweetened almond milk
1 teaspoon honey
½ cup plain nonfat Greek yogurt
½-1 teaspoon pure vanilla extract

Directions:
Pour coffee and almond milk into your blender. Add honey, yogurt, and vanilla extract. Blend until smooth.

Nutritional Info:
Total calories: 117
Carbs: 12.8
Fat: 2.6
Fiber: 0
Protein: 11.9

Cherry Latte Smoothie

Serves: 1

This 3-ingredient smoothie packs big flavors and nutrients for its simplicity. Cherries are an antioxidant powerhouse, and when combined with smooth cold brew and creamy almond milk, the flavor is irresistible. If you're used to really sweet coffees, add a little honey with the almond milk.

Ingredients:

½ cup unsweetened almond milk
½ cup cold brew coffee
¾ cup frozen cherries

Directions:

Pour milk and coffee into your blender. Add frozen cherries, then blend until smooth.

Nutritional Info:

Total calories: 81
Carbs: 15.2
Fat: 2.1
Fiber: 2.4
Protein: 1.8

A Berry Good Coffee Smoothie

Serves: 1

Antioxidant-rich berries and coffee go beautifully together. Have you ever enjoyed a mocha from a cafe with a shot of raspberry? This smoothie is inspired by that, though it uses frozen mixed berries. You can also use only your favorite berry if you want. For extra creaminess, we're using canned coconut milk.

Ingredients:

½ cup cold brew coffee

½ cup unsweetened coconut milk (from a can)

½ teaspoon vanilla

½ cup frozen berries

Directions:

Pour coffee and coconut milk into your blender. Add vanilla. Top with frozen berries, then blend until smooth.

Nutritional Info:

Total calories: 226

Carbs: 9

Fat: 18

Fiber: 1

Protein: 1

Mocha Smoothie (With Flaxseed)

Serves: 1

Mochas, which combine coffee and chocolate, are delicious when served iced. In this smoothie version, the mocha is made a bit healthier and protein-rich with Greek yogurt and ground flaxseed. Enjoy in the morning or as a treat on a hot day.

Ingredients:

½ cup unsweetened almond milk
½ cup cold brew coffee
1 teaspoon honey
½ cup plain nonfat Greek yogurt
½ teaspoon pure vanilla extract
1 tablespoon cocoa powder
1 tablespoon ground flaxseed

Directions:

Add almond milk, coffee, and honey to your blender. Scoop in yogurt, vanilla, cocoa powder, and ground flaxseed. Blend until smooth.

Nutritional Info:

Total calories: 162
Carbs: 22.5
Fat: 4.7
Fiber: 5.5
Protein: 9

Shot In the Dark Smoothie

Serves: 1

This protein-rich smoothie is perfect for lovers of espresso. Your normal morning shot is blended with almond milk, yogurt, cocoa powder, chia seeds, and a banana for sweetness. If you've never made chilled espresso before, just brew like normal, and pour over ice. Shake to cool.

Ingredients:

1 cup unsweetened almond milk

Shot of chilled espresso (about 1 ounce)

⅔ cup plain nonfat Greek yogurt

1 tablespoon cocoa powder

1 tablespoon of chia seeds

½ small frozen banana

Directions:

Pour milk and chilled espresso shot into your blender. Add yogurt, cocoa powder, and chia seeds. Top with frozen banana. Blend until smooth.

Nutritional Info:

Total calories: 242

Carbs: 36.5

Fat: 9.4

Fiber: 10.9

Protein: 13.6

Green Coffee Smoothie

Serves: 1

Trying to get more antioxidant-rich greens into your diet? Coffee is a great way to mask the Swiss chard (or spinach or kale) because of its strong flavor. Almond milk, honey, and banana add sweetness and balance to the smoothie, which is a perfect way to start the day or rejuvenate yourself in the middle of a long day.

Ingredients:

⅔ cup cold brew coffee
½ cup unsweetened almond milk
1 teaspoon honey
1 cup Swiss chard
½ small frozen banana

Directions:

Pour coffee and almond milk into your blender. Add honey, Swiss chard, and frozen banana. Blend until smooth.

Nutritional Info:

Total calories: 94
Carbs: 19.7
Fat: 2
Fiber: 2.4
Protein: 1.9

Hazelnut-Coffee Smoothie

Serves: 1

Hazelnut is a classic flavor addition to coffee. In this recipe, you can soak the hazelnuts overnight to improve their digestibility, but it isn't required. Soaking in warm water and a little salt can also improve the nutritional value. If you forget and still want to make this smoothie, go ahead. It will still be full of anti-cancer nutrients and delicious. Instead of a banana, we're using a more neutral-flavored alternative - an avocado - for thickness, fiber, potassium, and its other nutrients.

Tip: *If you really want to lean into the hazelnut, you can find hazelnut milk from brands like Pacific Foods.*

Ingredients:

½ cup unsweetened almond milk

½ cup cold brew coffee

1 teaspoon honey

¼ cup soaked hazelnuts

½ avocado

Directions:

Pour almond milk and coffee into your blender. Add honey, nuts, and avocado. Blend until smooth.

Nutritional Info:

Total calories: 427

Carbs: 20.2

Fat: 38.8

Fiber: 10

Protein: 6.9

Almond Butter Latte Smoothie

Serves: 1

In this smoothie, you're blending creamy almond butter, almond milk, and coffee together for a rich, nutty smoothie. Any nut butter will work, so feel free to experiment. For some omega-3 fatty acids and anti-inflammatory nutrients, we're also including ground flaxseed, which fits with the toasty flavor of this latte smoothie.

Ingredients:

½ cup unsweetened almond milk
½ cup cold brew coffee
½ teaspoon pure vanilla extract
1 tablespoon almond butter
1 tablespoon ground flaxseed
1 small frozen banana

Directions:

Pour milk, coffee, and vanilla into your blender. Add almond butter, flaxseed, and frozen banana. Blend until smooth.

Nutritional Info:

Total calories: 252
Carbs: 29.3
Fat: 13.3
Fiber: 6.6
Protein: 6.4

Mexican Coffee Smoothie

Serves: 1

Spiced with cinnamon and cayenne, this smoothie will wake you right up on sleepy mornings or early afternoons. Simply mix cold brew coffee with almond milk in a blender, and add spices. The frozen banana adds sweetness and thickens the drink. If you really like the cinnamon or cayenne, feel free to add more.

Ingredients:
½ cup unsweetened almond milk
½ cup cold brew coffee
½ teaspoon cinnamon
¼ teaspoon cayenne pepper
1 small frozen banana

Directions:
Pour milk and coffee into your blender. Add spices and banana. Blend until smooth.

Nutritional Info:
Total calories: 111
Carbs: 24.1
Fat: 2.1
Fiber: 3.1
Protein: 1.7

Pumpkin Spice Latte Smoothie

Serves: 1

When fall rolls around, pumpkin spice lattes take over. In this smoothie version, we're actually adding some real pumpkin in the form of antioxidant-rich pumpkin seeds. All the spices are represented, too - cinnamon, ginger, and nutmeg. For sweetness, mix in a little honey.

Ingredients:
½ cup unsweetened almond milk
½ cup cold brew coffee
½ tablespoon honey
1 tablespoon ground pumpkin seeds
1 teaspoon cinnamon
¼ teaspoon ground ginger
¼ teaspoon ground nutmeg
1 small frozen banana

Directions:
Pour almond milk and coffee in your blender. Add honey, ground pumpkin seeds, and spices. Top with frozen banana. Blend until smooth.

Nutritional Info:
Total calories: 190
Carbs: 34.3
Fat: 6.1
Fiber: 3.5
Protein: 3.9

Peppermint Latte Smoothie

Serves: 1

Peppermint lattes are often served hot and during the winter, but if you're craving a little Christmas time in the summer, this is a great smoothie. You can make it any time of year, however, there are no rules. Simply blend almond milk, Greek yogurt, cold brew coffee, peppermint extract, and a frozen banana together.

Tip: *Turn this into a peppermint **mocha** smoothie by adding 1 tablespoon of cocoa powder.*

Ingredients:
¼ cup unsweetened almond milk
¼ cup nonfat plain Greek yogurt
½ cup cold brew coffee
⅛ teaspoon peppermint extract
1 small frozen banana

Directions:
Pour almond milk, yogurt, and coffee into your blender. Add peppermint and frozen banana. Blend until smooth.

Nutritional Info:
Total calories: 134
Carbs: 28.8
Fat: 1.2
Fiber: 3.6
Protein: 4.5

Vietnamese Coffee Smoothie (With Chia Seeds)

Serves: 1

Vietnamese coffee is defined by sweetened condensed milk and strong coffee, so in this recipe, we're actually using the undiluted concentrate. It gets blended with coconut milk and sweetened condensed milk for a rich, creamy taste. For some nutrients with anti-cancer properties, we're adding chia seeds.

Ingredients:

½ cup unsweetened coconut milk (from a carton)
½ cup cold brew coffee concentrate (not diluted)
2 teaspoons sweetened condensed milk
1 tablespoon of chia seeds
½ small frozen banana

Directions:

Pour coconut milk, coffee, and sweetened condensed milk into your blender. Add chia seeds and frozen banana. Blend until smooth.

Nutritional Info:

Total calories: 190
Carbs: 28
Fat: 10.3
Fiber: 7.3
Protein: 4.6

Almond Joy Coffee Smoothie

Serves: 1

Almond Joy bars are probably my favorite candy. In this coffee smoothie, you get the coconut from coconut milk and coconut extract, which you can easily find with the vanilla in the store. Grind the almonds and flaxseed together for convenience; together, they add fiber and cancer-fighting nutrients. Top smoothie with a few ice cubes for thickness and a nice chill.

Ingredients:

1 cup unsweetened coconut milk (from a carton)

½ cup cold brew coffee

½ teaspoon coconut extract

2 tablespoons ground almonds

½ tablespoon ground flaxseed

Couple of ice cubes

Directions:

Pour milk, coffee, and coconut extract into your blender. Add ground almonds and flaxseed. Top with a few ice cubes. Blend until smooth.

Nutritional Info:

Total calories: 133

Carbs: 5.6

Fat: 11.1

Fiber: 3.4

Protein: 3.3

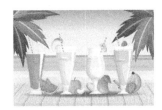

Chapter 11: Dessert Smoothies (Cancer Prevention + During Treatment)

While labeled as "dessert," these recipes still contain lots of healthy ingredients that are part of a diet that fights cancer or the side effects of cancer treatment. You'll see nonfat Greek yogurt, berries, chia seeds, and more. I've also tried to rely mostly on the natural sweetness of fruit, so you won't see a lot of refined sweeteners. If you're looking for better dessert alternatives with ingredients that might prevent cancer, or higher-calorie smoothies during your cancer treatment, these are the ones to make.

Chocolate-Covered Berry Smoothie

Apple Pie Smoothie

Cookies + Cream Smoothie

Black Forest Smoothie

Sunbutter-Oatmeal Cookie Smoothie

Lemon-Coconut Bar Smoothie

Key Lime Pie Smoothie

Chocolate-Covered Cashew Smoothie

Carrot Cake Smoothie

Secret Ingredient Chocolate Smoothie

Chocolate-Covered Berry Smoothie

Serves: 1

Chocolate-covered strawberries are a great gift on Valentine's Day, and in this smoothie, you're adding raspberries to the list. The two fruits together are more interesting and go great with almond milk, nonfat Greek yogurt, and of course, cocoa powder. For some extra nutrients, you're adding chia seeds, too. Double the servings for a Valentine's Day treat or dessert on date night.

Ingredients:
- 1 cup unsweetened almond milk
- ¼ cup nonfat Greek yogurt
- ½ tablespoon of chia seeds
- 1 tablespoon unsweetened dark cocoa powder
- ½ cup frozen strawberries
- ½ cup frozen raspberries

Directions:
Pour almond milk into your blender. Add yogurt, chia seeds, and dark cocoa powder. Top with frozen berries. Blend until smooth.

Nutritional Info:
- Total calories: 170
- Carbs: 25
- Fat: 6
- Fiber: 8
- Protein: 8

Apple Pie Smoothie

Serves: 1

The all-American apple pie is very easy to make in smoothie form. All you need is almond milk, some spices, an apple, and a frozen banana for sweetness and texture. Choose your apple based on how sweet you like your pie (or smoothie). A green apple will be a lot tarter, while apples like Honeycrisp and Gala have more sugar. If you're increasing the servings of this smoothie to make enough for friends and family, you could also use a combination of sweet and tart apples. The blend will make for a delicious and interesting flavor profile.

Ingredients:

    1 cup unsweetened almond milk
    1 teaspoon ground cinnamon
    Pinch of nutmeg
    Pinch of ground ginger
    1 chopped apple
    ½ frozen banana

Directions:

Pour almond milk into your blender. Add spices, apple, and then top with frozen banana. Blend until smooth.

Nutritional Info:

    Total calories: 209
    Carbs: 46.3
    Fat: 4.1
    Fiber: 7.9
    Protein: 2.2

Cookies + Cream Smoothie

Serves: 1

A classic milkshake, I've made cookies + cream a little better for you with almond milk, nonfat Greek yogurt, Oreos, vanilla, and a banana. It is far less sweet than anything you'd buy at an ice cream shop, but still rich and delicious as a treat on a summer day.

Ingredients:

1 cup unsweetened almond milk

½ cup plain nonfat Greek yogurt

4 crushed Oreo cookies

½ teaspoon vanilla extract

½ frozen banana

Directions:

Pour milk and yogurt into your blender. Add cookies, vanilla, and frozen banana. Blend until smooth.

Nutritional Info:

Total calories: 348

Carbs: 47

Fat: 14

Fiber: 1

Protein: 10

Black Forest Smoothie

Serves: 1

Cherry and chocolate get married in this smoothie inspired by Black Forest cake, a German dessert made with chocolate sponge, whipped cream, and cherries. We've made that a bit healthier with almond milk and vanilla extract, cocoa powder, cherries, and chia seeds. If you really love chocolate, this is a great dessert smoothie.

Ingredients:
1 cup unsweetened almond milk
½ teaspoon vanilla extract
1 tablespoon cocoa powder
1 tablespoon of chia seeds
½ cup fresh or frozen pitted cherries
½ frozen banana

Directions:
Pour milk and vanilla extract into your blender. Add cocoa powder, chia seeds, cherries, and the banana half. Blend until smooth.

Nutritional Info:
Total calories: 218
Carbs: 36.9
Fat: 9.9
Fiber: 10.6
Protein: 6.1

Sunbutter-Oatmeal Cookie Smoothie

Serves: 1

This smoothie is technically cold, but it's full of warm flavors like honey, oats, sunflower butter, and cinnamon. If you find yourself craving a cookie, but don't want to make a batch, make this smoothie instead. As well as being tasty, sunflower seeds are full of antioxidants, so this is a good treat to make if you're looking for ingredients that lower your risk for cancer.

Ingredients:

1 cup unsweetened almond milk

½ teaspoon vanilla extract

½ tablespoon honey

1 tablespoon sunflower butter

3 tablespoons oats

½ frozen banana

Pinch of cinnamon

Directions:

Pour milk and vanilla into your blender. Add honey, sunflower butter, and oats. Lastly, add banana. Blend until smooth. Sprinkle with cinnamon before enjoying.

Nutritional Info:

Total calories: 275

Carbs: 38.9

Fat: 12.3

Fiber: 4.1

Protein: 6.8

Lemon-Coconut Bar Smoothie

Serves: 1

Lemon and coconut are a great flavor combination. The tropical sweetness of coconut balances out the sharp sourness of the lemon. In this smoothie, the coconut comes from milk and a teeny bit of coconut extract. For the lemon, all you need is fresh lemon juice and, if you want, some lemon zest on top. This is a great dessert smoothie when you want something light, fresh, and clean-tasting.

Ingredients:

½ cup unsweetened coconut milk (from a carton)
½ teaspoon coconut extract
¼ cup plain nonfat Greek yogurt
2 tablespoons fresh lemon juice
1 frozen banana
Sprinkle of lemon zest (optional)

Directions:

Pour milk and coconut extract into your blender. Add nonfat Greek yogurt, lemon juice, and frozen banana. Blend until smooth. If desired, top with a sprinkle of lemon zest.

Nutritional Info:

Total calories: 222
Carbs: 33.1
Fat: 9.1
Fiber: 4.2
Protein: 3.8

Key Lime Pie Smoothie

Serves: 1

Is there anything quite as refreshing as a slice of key lime pie? This smoothie embraces those flavors, with flaxseed replacing graham crackers for some extra health benefits. If you're worried that the almond milk and banana will overpower the lime, never fear, because lime comes from two sources - lime yogurt *and* fresh lime juice. The bright, citrusy flavor is unmistakable.

Tip: Lime yogurt

You can find quite a few lime-flavored yogurts on the market. Fage, Dannon Oikos, and Chobani all make key lime yogurts. The Fage actually comes separated, with the key lime jelly in a separate container. All three have roughly the same amount of sugar and protein.

Ingredients:
    1 cup unsweetened almond milk
    1 teaspoon honey
    ¼ cup lime-flavored yogurt
    1 tablespoon fresh lime juice
    ½ tablespoon ground flaxseed
    ½ frozen banana

Directions:
Pour milk, honey, yogurt, and lime juice into your blender. Add flaxseed and banana. Blend until smooth.

Nutritional Info:
    Total calories: 214
    Carbs: 31.4
    Fat: 7
    Fiber: 3.5
    Protein: 7.8

Chocolate-Covered Cashew Smoothie

Serves: 1

You've heard of chocolate-covered almonds, which are popular around Christmas, but in this smoothie, you're replacing almonds with cashews. These fatty, tasty nuts add a mild flavor to the smoothie, so if you aren't usually a fan of nuts, you probably won't notice them. The flavor of rich cocoa powder, sweet honey, and creamy almond milk will be stronger.

Ingredients:

1 cup unsweetened almond milk
½ tablespoon honey
1 tablespoon cocoa powder
½ cup ground cashews
½ frozen banana

Directions:

Pour milk into your blender. Add honey, cocoa powder, and ground cashews. Top with frozen banana. Blend until smooth.

Nutritional Info:

Total calories: 530
Carbs: 49.5
Fat: 36.2
Fiber: 6.2
Protein: 13.1

Carrot Cake Smoothie

Serves: 1

Sweet and spiced, carrot cake is a comforting classic. In this smoothie version, we're using coconut milk, plenty of carrots, and spices. For sweetener, it's maple syrup and a banana, which also helps with the thickness. Carrots are full of nutrients like beta-carotene, while cinnamon and ginger have anti-inflammatory properties.

Ingredients:
    1 cup unsweetened coconut milk (from a carton)
    ½ cup plain nonfat Greek yogurt
    2 teaspoons maple syrup
    1 cup diced carrots
    Pinch of cinnamon
    Pinch of ground ginger
    ½ frozen banana

Directions:
Pour the cup of milk into the blender and add Greek yogurt and maple syrup. Add carrots, spices, and banana. Blend until smooth.

Nutritional Info:
    Total calories: 242
    Carbs: 45.7
    Fat: 4.2
    Fiber: 6.7
    Protein: 7.5

Secret Ingredient Chocolate Smoothie

Serves: 1

With just four ingredients, this chocolate smoothie is very easy to make. What's the secret ingredient? Cooked chickpeas, also known as garbanzo beans. They add thickness and anti-cancer ingredients like protein, fiber, and phytochemicals, but you won't taste them at all thanks to the rich cocoa powder and sweet banana. This is a completely guilt-free dessert.

Ingredients:

    1 cup unsweetened almond milk
    1 tablespoon cocoa powder
    ¼ cup cooked chickpeas
    1 small frozen banana

Directions:

Pour milk into your blender. Add cocoa powder, chickpeas, and banana. Blend until smooth.

Nutritional Info:

    Total calories: 213
    Carbs: 41.6
    Fat: 5.2
    Fiber: 7.9
    Protein: 6.1

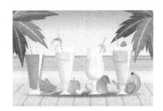

Epilogue

Nutrition, nutrition, nutrition. It's a word (along with "nutrients") you've seen a lot in this book, so you know by now how important it is. Cancer can manifest for a variety of reasons, and sometimes there's nothing we can do to stop it, but studies keep showing that good nutrition is one of the best ways to reduce the risk. Research also shows that good nutrition *during* cancer and during the resulting treatment is essential. That's why this book has smoothies for both cancer prevention and during treatment, because there is no magic formula guaranteed to stop the disease from happening. Of course, that doesn't mean you should stop eating healthy, and my hope is that you add smoothies to your diet as an easy way to get more good nutrition in your life.

How do you do that? The first step: get a blender. In chapter 3, I broke down everything you need to consider when shopping, including the blender's power, blades, jug, price, and additional features. With a good blender, you'll be able to make all the smoothies in this book and thoroughly blend in ingredients like carrots, frozen fruit, protein powder, and so on. Be sure to stock up on freezer bags, ice cube trays, and consider getting a food processor for nuts, nut butter, and oats.

What ingredients should go into that blender? In chapter 1, I walked through a handful of the ingredients that come up frequently, like berries, dark leafy greens, chia seeds, cinnamon, honey, tea, and Greek yogurt. These are by no means the *only* anti-cancer ingredients out there, and as you do other research and make smoothies beyond these recipes, you'll discover more. The list just gives you an idea of the types of nutrients and food researchers have been looking at over the last decades.

Hopefully, you feel more confident in your knowledge about anti-cancer nutrition and how to get those nutrients through smoothies. Even more than that, however, I hope you now believe that *all* smoothies (yes, even green ones) can be as delicious as they are nutritious. I understand that lots of "health" food is often code for "food that doesn't taste good," but that doesn't have to be the case. While a lot of the recipes in this book could probably have more nutrients packed in with different additions, or more of a certain ingredient, it would affect the taste, and if you don't like a smoothie, you're not going to keep making it. I think we would all be okay sacrificing small amounts of nutrients for the sake of getting those nutrients at all.

Made in the USA
Las Vegas, NV
29 October 2024

10721258R00079